Art as Therapy

Art as Therapy

Inspiration, Innovation, and Ideas

Diane Fausek-Steinbach

Idyll Arbor, Inc.

PO Box 720, Ravensdale, WA 98051 (360) 825-7797

Idyll Arbor, Inc. Editor: Thomas M. Blaschko

To the best of our knowledge, the information and recommendations of this book reflect currently accepted practice. Nevertheless, they cannot be considered absolute and universal. Recommendations for a particular client must be considered in light of the client's needs and condition. The author and publisher disclaim responsibility for any adverse effects resulting directly or indirectly from the suggested practices, from any undetected errors, or from the reader's misunderstanding of the text.

Library of Congress Cataloging-in-Publication Data

Fausek-Steinbach, Diane, 1963-

Art as therapy : inspiration, innovation, and ideas / Diane Fausek-Steinbach.

p. ; cm.

Includes bibliographical references and index.

ISBN-13: 978-1-882883-57-8 (alk. paper)

ISBN-10: 1-882883-57-8 (alk. paper)

1. Art therapy. I. Title.

[DNLM: 1. Art Therapy--methods. 2. Mental Disorders--therapy.
WM 450.5.A8 F267a 2005]

RC489.A7F37 2005

616.89'1656--dc22

2005019356

ISBN 978-1-882883-57-8
ISBN 1-882883-57-8

For Sandy

Lifelong friend.
Thank you for helping to shape all the good things that I am,
and for overlooking all the less-than-good things, for over 30 years.

and

For Norman

Lifelong love…

Contents

Art Projects

Table of Illustrations

Chapter 1

Introduction

Art is a powerful weapon that can be used against many enemies: lack of communication, solitude, depression, and confusion. Art can be used as a creative approach to deal with issues such as control, loss, forgiveness, self-esteem, reality orientation, and socialization. It can help reach therapeutic goals for persons of all ages and abilities. The right art materials along with clear directives and a well thought out plan can open doors within clients and revitalize their lives. It is an important skill that you can develop and use with almost any population, or in dealing with your own issues. Knowing the risks, the mechanics, and the possibilities can help you bring the use of art as therapy to those you seek to help.

The purpose of this book is to give you an understanding of the responsibilities and potentials of using art as therapy, some practical advice on utilizing your unique interests and talents to enhance your groups, and a running start with group plans to challenge clients of all abilities.

I will also discuss the future of art as therapy, with a look at modern technology and how it can help you connect your clients with exciting new possibilities.

Common Sense: Know the Dangers and Risks

Using art materials with a variety of cognitive and physically functioning clients can be challenging. There are some simple rules to think about when preparing a group or creating a plan.

Spoons are for the Kitchen

When working in a residential or institutional setting it's easy to grab the ready resources to get your group going. Using plastic spoons to stir or dispense paints is quick and easy; no clean up or initial expenses are required. However, you must think about the skills and cognitive abilities of your group members. If there is one forgetful person in your group, or just one person with a modified mental status, using a spoon (or any other kitchen utensil) in the production of your artwork is potentially hazardous.

I ran an art studio where I had clients of all abilities coming and going from my art room, working on different projects. My client, Doris (not her real name), had suffered a stroke, but seemed oriented and alert during the process of art making. I turned away from her to address another client, while she busily worked on a ceramic piece. When I turned back to face her, she was licking the paintbrush off as if it were a spoon coming out of cookie batter. I called her name, and we both were surprised to find her with a mouth full of ceramic paint. She was daydreaming and forgot what she was doing. Now, that happened while she was using appropriate art tools (the paintbrush). Think of how confusing it might be for clients who are forgetful or who have dementia to suddenly find themselves with a spoon in their hand. Avoid disaster. Invest in appropriate art tools when working with clients.

Safety First

If you are working with clients with violent tendencies or unpredictable behavior, consider the safety of the art materials you are using. For example, if I am working with clients who are paranoid or have shown confrontational behavior in the past, I may want additional help in my art group to monitor items like scissors or other sharp implements. I would not use nature materials like rocks with violent teens, and I would not plan an art process that might excite and energize a dangerous population unless there is ample follow-up time for the group to decompress and calm down. Find alternative materials (for instance, use papier-mâché rocks for a project) or reconsider the process. If you are unsure, always take the safe ground.

Always use Non-Toxic Materials

These days most art materials are non-toxic or have a non-toxic alternative. Even if it is a bit more expensive, opt for the safer material. Also, request Material Safety Data Sheets (MSDS) in case something should happen and you need to give an EMT or nurse additional information on the products that you are using. When ordering your art materials, simply ask that these sheets be included in the packaging, or write the manufacturer.

Chapter 2

Working Together

Incorporating different modalities into your art group can breathe new life into your program just when you may be running out of ideas. Music and recreational therapy are just two possible realms you may want to explore.

Music therapy is a creative means of using the appeal of music, instrument utilization, music education, and other musical interventions to help people of all ages and all abilities.

Recreational therapy utilizes structured activities as a form of treatment. It is successful and widely used in all institutional settings. If you are lucky enough to have these professionals at your facility or in your department, brainstorm ways to work together for the betterment of your clients. I have often worked with music therapists with a variety of client populations and have found the collaboration to be mutually beneficial. With fully functioning, high cognitive level clients, music therapy can be used as an inspiration for abstract art. With more challenging clients it can be part of an art/music/sensory stimulation program based on a theme.

For instance, ask a music therapist to introduce your group to a type of music they may not have experienced before. Explore the background of the artist, or the culture, then step in and ask the group to creatively express their understanding through paints or oil pastels. With lower functioning clients, promote the use of simple rhythm instruments and then imitate the movements by hitting clay in rhythm to create design.

With recreational therapists, you can create and implement original trivia games or movement games where art materials may be incorporated. Create a game based on color or shape identification for your lower level clients, or design an activity around an artistic style for your higher level clients.

Your art group doesn't always have to have art media as the spotlight, and doesn't always have to show results in displayable art. It is the action, the understanding, and the challenge of the process that provides the most benefits.

Another way to work together with others in your facility is to utilize your finished art pieces as stimulation for others in the environment. When appropriate, and with the agreement of the artists, display art work in community locations and encourage support staff to use it as a point of conversation with confused or withdrawn clients. Let people know that there is a great opportunity to stimulate the senses by exposing others in the population to the vibrant, expressive, and (sometimes) texturally interesting work your group is doing. Display your group members' work with information on what the process or theme was, provide material information, and even suggest conversation starters. By doing this you are initiating an interdisciplinary approach to the socialization issues in your facility, and may even inspire new clients to join the fun!

Finally, working together means utilizing your human resources. Take advantage of a volunteer program at your facility and request art students or retired individuals with artistic skills. Preparation is sometimes necessary for unique art plans, and free time is usually at a minimum. A skilled sewer could save you time by finishing off quilted murals or other fabric projects. Perhaps there are a few family members who would love to spend part of their visit with their loved one cutting out magazine photos for future collage work. Getting to know your local human resources and planning ahead can make your world a lot easier.

Don't forget to introduce yourself to the local college art instructors or art therapy program directors. Perhaps they can add your facility to their placement list for potential experiential sites for their students. Anywhere you can find an extra hand or two can only make your group run more smoothly, be more safe, and allow for more one-to-one communication with your clients.

Chapter 3

Thinking Creatively

Creating original and interesting art plans takes time. You need to invest in discovering and appreciating different aspects of everyday life. See what is around you with a discerning eye and determine how you can apply your own interests and experiences to your work. Here are a few pointers to get you started.

Broaden Your Horizons

Challenge yourself to learn new things, to open new books, to look at everything you see, hear, taste, and touch with an art process in mind. Think about issues that your clients may be dealing with and try to apply those issues to art media. Look at history books and study the illustrations. Get a magnifying glass and dissect how they were drawn. Can you replicate that somehow? Read stories, myths, and lore. Study the illustrations; think about the story's focus. Does it hold a lesson for you that you can pass on?

For example, in the lesson plan "Instruments of Communication" from my book *Art Activities for Groups. Providing Therapy, Fun and Function* (Idyll Arbor, 2002), the plan was to make a basic rattling instrument, but it was based upon a Norse myth about a watchman that couldn't speak. The story's focus was on how he communicated without talking. I took that theme and focused my plan around how clients may not always say what they mean, or may have other communication issues. Relating the process to a piece of literature made the process age-appropriate, inspiring, and non-threatening. It gave clients an opportunity to be creative and open a discussion about their own communication challenges.

Open up an art history or modern art book. Modern abstract art holds a lot of inspiration for processes you could do with your clients. Bringing a sample of well-known abstract or "Pop" art could make an art process seem less threatening and encourage those hesitant artists to just "give it a try." For example, I used the works of Kandinsky and Rothko as inspiration for the "Variation of 12" plan (page 76) and "Rothko Inspired Pastels" (page 79) to inspire art creation and teach a little art history as well! Check out the works of Klee and Whatmore also for more great examples of beautiful and well-known art work that your clients may be able to recreate or gain inspiration from.

Another inspirational source I use is architecture and statuary. The familiar shapes of well-known buildings or even bridges may strike you with line and detail when you look at it with an artistic eye. Forget about what the object itself is and look at it as shapes, textures, and colors. Can you apply those shapes to a collage project or mural? A closer look at local statuary that you may find outside of your courthouse or as part of downtown monuments or displays may rouse some new ideas about working with nature objects, such as stone or clay.

Narrow Your Focus

Now that you have expanded your experiential palette, it is time to take another look at life on a microscopic level. Your perception of how beautiful things are depends on your ability to see and focus. Do you appreciate the tonal color qualities of an ant as we walk by it on the sidewalk? How does a drop of water reflect light and color? Investigate amoebas and scientific elements through a microscope. The publication, "Molecular Expressions: Microscopy Publications — Fabrications of Unusual Art Forms" (www.micro.magnet.fsu.edu/publications/pages/microscope.html), has impressive imagery of various elements to get you on your way, and was the inspiration for my plan "Fantasy Landscapes" (page 45.)

Think of how you can magnify common elements of your daily lives and focus on their folds, their sharp edges. Even a closer look at the palm of your hand can be a beautiful beginning to an art plan.

There are many ways to get microscopic views of nature and science: through the Internet, science books or magazines, and other library resources. Don't be afraid to just isolate and enlarge everyday objects on a copy machine, such as plant foliage, fringe from a pillow, or feathers, for use in a collage or painting project.

Find Inspiration in the Words of Others

Loss, friendship, love, and family are all common issues your clients may be dealing with. Research inspirational quotes related to these topics and incorporate them into an art project. Let a poet, civil rights leader, movie star, or famous author provide a launching point for painting. Let them open the door to further discussion of the issues your clients find important, and (all too frequently) under dialogued. There are many books available highlighting familiar or theme related quotations. Books such as *Chicken Soup for the Soul* (Canfield Health Communications, 1999) and *The Enduring Human Spirit* (Idyll Arbor, 2003) may contain stories that you may be able to use to inspire creativity in your group.

Use Guided Imagery and Story Exercises

Imagery can be used to help people achieve a variety of goals. A trained guided imagery specialist uses his/her knowledge to help people deal with anxiety or depression, overcome phobias, relax, and heal. In art therapy, guided imagery (or as I use it, modified guided story exercises) can encourage clients to use their imaginations to create original artwork.

To begin, you may want to set the mood with quiet music and a soft voice, then allow your high functioning clients to immerse themselves in a safe and warm, imaginative place. There is a section in chapter 5 that delves into guided stories and their uses. One must use this type of guided imagery responsibly however, as it could be unsettling to clients who are confused or disoriented. Use it only with high functioning clients with no mental illness or instability. Consult a trained guided imagery specialist and work together if possible!

Recycle and Rework

We don't always have time to reinvent the wheel. Sometimes a quick yet purposeful group idea is needed. Think back on previous projects you have done, or revisit some of projects detailed in this book. Can you rework this process by changing the theme or the media? Adapting one idea to meet the needs of clients of all different cognitive and physical functioning levels can be done easily if you plan for additional help during the group process, or spend more time preparing materials prior to the group start time. Trying out a plan yourself may take some time, but it generally saves time later by providing you that extra bit of information on additional material needs and mess prevention. It also allows time to troubleshoot potentially frustrating elements of the plan. Your ultimate goal is to make your art group hassle-free for your clients, so that they can focus on the creative elements rather than the mechanical ones.

Chapter 4

Utilizing New Technology and the Internet

Modern technology has thrown the doors wide open in the world of art. New imaging equipment can create exciting new opportunities to an artist and lots of inspiration for creativity to a therapist. Matching and adapting the new technology with your clients' needs must be done very carefully. You need to consider both the benefits and challenges of teaching and learning new techniques using modern equipment, and determine how much preparation and intervention needs to be done in order to ensure a successful and exciting process.

Some technology is relatively easy to learn, while others may have too many steps involved to make it a realistic plan for your population. Also, modern equipment, such as digital cameras, scanners, and computer programs cost money. Most facilities will not make an investment of this sort for your art groups. However, chances are if you work in a moderately sized facility, somebody in some department has what you need and would be willing to let you utilize it from time to time. Talk to the other staff in your facility. Make a request in your newsletter or volunteer department for equipment donations or loans.

Digital Cameras

Digital cameras are great to use during one-to-one or small group programs. With higher level cognitive function clients, you can begin a class on basic photography, taking turns using the camera and setting up artistic shots of foliage or other matters of interest, which can be printed out later by you for further use in collage or paintings.

Challenge your clients to take ten minutes and find five examples of things that make them happy, sad, or bring back childhood memories and take pictures of them. Taking turns with the camera, each artist would take pictures you can later print out and display. This could also be done with an instant camera, however you are then limited to a small final image. Compared to a standard camera or even disposable camera, the digital camera allows for quick image turnaround and instant gratification for the artist.

When buying a digital camera, remember that resolution is pretty much everything, so buy one with zoom capabilities and the most megapixels you can afford. (Four is usually sufficient.)

Scanners

Having a scanner attached to a computer in your activity area will allow you to create the same type of artwork you could do using items copied on a standard copy machine. For example, "Fantasy Landscapes" in the collage chapter of this book was done with images copied or scanned from their original source. Scanning usually gives you an option of color images that, when coupled with a color printer, can be valuable in collage creations. You can scan a variety of objects for collage use, or personalize a process by scanning client's family photos or mementos for later use in a collage process.

Color Copying

If you don't have a scanner or color printer, a trip to the local copy shop will usually provide you with the ability to make color copies. Again, color copies are a great way to create unique and original images to be used in a collage process. Colors will usually be more vibrant than if an image is hand colored with pencils or paints, and will allow the artist to see the collage materials as part of a color scheme, rather than just an image with texture or shape.

Computer Programs for One-on-One Art

The use of art programs like PC Paintbrush or Adobe Photoshop can allow high level clients who may have limited mobility or range of motion to create exciting artwork with small moves of a mouse and clicks of a button. Again, you must be able to spend time with the client to show them how to use the basic components of the programs, so it is most effective with rehabilitative clients on a one-to-one basis. Teaching clients how to manipulate images through the computer can also help break someone out of depression by giving them something exciting to work on, stimulating their intellect by using modern technology, and making them feel more part of the world around them. Pair up an interested client with a computer savvy volunteer and let them explore.

Take a client's digital or scanned photo and show how to experiment with the many artistic filters available in the Adobe Photoshop program. This is a quick and relatively easy process that can excite the imagination of even your most uninvolved or anti-social clients. Seeing their original image transformed into a watercolor painting, or covered in cyber plastic wrap may inspire them to create an Andy Warhol-like mural or to make personalized greeting cards for family and friends.

The Internet

Utilize the Internet to research art techniques, unique artists, and historical information to share with your clients. Many of the projects in this book refer to Internet sites or reference well-known artists that you can research to show your clients the potentials of different art media. I use the Internet as a point of inspiration for planning art groups. Sometimes I can find web sites that offer high resolution (hi res.) images that I can then print out and use for collage work or reference for paintings or drawings.

Here are just a few sites I have used for inspiration or reference. Some sites are tied to art supply companies or businesses, which you may further investigate if you wish. Their inclusion here does not indicate any specific endorsement on my part, or on the part of the publisher.

Web pages move and links are broken at times. If you have problems accessing the sites listed here, try doing a search using words from the original website name, or search under words listed in the description area. All sites were viable at the time of publication.

Basic art education sites

http://www.artcyclopedia.com/ This is a great site for browsing art images and includes lots of links to art museum web sites.

http://www.askart.com/ Nice listing of well known artists with examples of their work and links to other sites and image galleries.

http://www.crayola.com/educators/techniques Some fun techniques and instructions to use with Crayola products.

http://www.sanford-artedventures.com/create/create.html Nice site with some creative ideas that you can adapt to suit your population.

http://www.watchingpaintdry.com Click on the "Techniques and Tips" section for some ideas on painting lesson plans as well as other art ideas. Also links to further articles in *Artist's Magazine.*

https://www.saxarts.com/index.jsp Has lesson plans and product tips that you can adapt for your own population. Also lots of information for the novice artist regarding supplies and maintenance of your valuable materials.

http://www.kstrom.net/isk/art/art.html Information about Native American art, especially from the Great Plains; links to many other sites.

http://www.northwest-art.com/ Samples of art from the natives of the Pacific Northwest.

http://www.liunet.edu/cwis/cwp/library/aavaahp.htm The C.W. Post Campus display of African American art.

http://artarchives.si.edu/guides/ The Smithsonian's Archives of American Art with information about the art of several of the cultures in North America including Latino, Asian American, and African American.

http://www.stampin.com Nice site if you are a rubber stamping enthusiast. If you are not, check out the "templates" section, which you could use with other media!

http://www.meininger.com Check out the "Education Center" portion of the website. "Tips and Techniques" has some good advice for novice artists including some answers to common questions with a variety of media types. Also, take a look at the "Lesson Plans" area for inspiration on ideas you may be able to use with your population.

http://www.homecrafts.co.uk/index.asp Go to the "Techniques" area for great information on basic arts and crafts instruction. You can also download with Adobe Acrobat, PDF files with detailed instruction on art plans such as how to make decorative fabric boxes or greeting cards.

http://www.gsdye.com/Canada/instructional_sheets.html Nice website with information on a variety of fabric dying techniques including tie dying. Great ideas under "Microwave Scarf dying."

http://www.coxes.com/muse/2000-05/jo/ Good information on collage as an art form with many links for further exploration.

http://www.origami.as/home.html Interesting information on Origami, including instructions for novice and experienced paper folders.

http://www.creativity-portal.com Check out the "How To" directory for lots of links and instructions for common art processes.

http://drawsketch.about.com/library/blintro.htm?PM=ss11_drawsketch Basic information on drawing skills. Great for the inexperienced.

Cultural arts sites

http://www.theartofafrica.co.za/africa/index.jsp Nice website with lots of information on the history of African cultures. It has an interesting section on myths and folklore as well as some good information on traditional rock art techniques.

http://www.yale.edu/swahili/ The Kamusi Project Internet Living Swahili Dictionary; An interesting language site used for the "Bits of Africa" project on page 42.

http://www.asia-art.net/chinese_tech_brush.html Interesting website discussing the philosophy and basics of Chinese brush painting. Also has information on other Asian art forms. You may not be able to put it to practical use, but it has loads of educational value and images you may find inspirational.

http://www.geocities.com/ginis/ Cool Graphics. Has plenty of links to other free websites with photo images and graphics you can use. Includes NASA sites, arts and crafts sites, and more.

Inspirational sites

http://micro.magnet.fsu.edu/publications/pages/microscope.html Molecular Expressions: Microscopy Publications – Fabrications of Unusual Art Forms. This is a science website which investigates the use of molecular images as a base for creative expression. Browse around and you will find some really unusual artwork!

www.nasa.gov/home NASA website featuring breathtaking images from space. To access the Voyager and Galileo sections, use the search function. Browse through the entire site. Images are high resolution and can be downloaded easily.

http://www.spiritoftrees.org/folktales/folktales.html Interesting collection of stories about trees.

http://www.webshots.com/homepage.html Has high resolution photographs you can download and use for collage work or just for inspiration!

Chapter 5

Creating the Best Environment

Identifying an individual's challenges and strengths before placing them into an art group is important. You want to group together clients who have similar needs, issues and abilities so that you can create the most beneficial art experience for them. Clients who need more directions or hand-over-hand assistance should not be placed in a group of more independent clients because both populations may find it a frustrating and non-productive experience. Without labeling the individual, we do need to address differences in cognitive and physical functioning levels so that appropriate group preparation and implementation can take place.

For the purposes of this book I have broken down basic client skills into ***high, medium,*** and ***low*** level cognitive and physical functioning. These are broad categories that will be used to indicate a certain level of functioning needed to complete each process successfully. Success here is based on the client's level of satisfaction with the group, a positive experience (one that does not contribute to low self-esteem and builds a good self image), and opportunities to be creative or to reminisce.

The ***high*** level cognitive and physical functioning category (hereafter referred to as "high level") would address clients of the general population. This level includes persons who are in long term care or rehabilitation facilities, with good memory function or ability to handle multi-step processes. The ability to think abstractly and work independently or with adaptive utensils would also be included. They should show an interest in art and indicate a desire to participate in an art-based program. Groups at this level should include six to ten persons to ensure the opportunity for individual attention and therapeutic processing of images. You could offer an open art studio experience for this level clientele so that they might explore their own artistic interests, as well as a therapeutic art group to address common issues and concerns. Group times should be from 45 minutes for a structured group up to two hours for an art studio experience.

The ***medium*** level cognitive and physical functioning category (hereafter referred to as "medium level") includes clients with some minor forgetfulness and physical challenges. They should be able to work independently with limited assistance. They should be able to decide to come to group whether by invitation or reminder. Adaptive equipment and modified art plans can address mobility issues, but, generally, these group members should be motivated and should require minimal prompts to complete a process. Groups could be anywhere from four to eight persons, depending on the process, to ensure the ability to help clients as necessary without slowing down the progress of the whole group. This level client may also benefit from an open studio type program, where they can work at their own pace with some assistance or "starting points" offered by staff. A structured art as therapy group would also be beneficial and may focus on group cooperation and socialization in addition to challenging and stimulating the mind with a variety of art media and processes. Group times may be anywhere from 25 to 45 minutes, depending on the process.

The ***low*** level cognitive and physical functioning category (hereafter referred to as "low level") includes clients who have significant confusion or dementia, can use at least one hand, have the ability to follow one-step directions, and participate with some hand-over-hand assistance, if necessary. Work with these clients may focus on cognitive goals such as color or shape identification, reminiscence, and group interaction. Physical goals such as fine and gross motor skills and maintaining eye contact appropriately could also be addressed. Group numbers should be limited to four to six depending on materials. These programs are sensory in focus with the emphasis being on the process and not on a "completed art piece." Average group time would be shorter, perhaps 15 to 20 minutes, to address a shorter attention span. Art materials might be limited to collage media and fabric processes to capitalize on the sensory opportunities and maximize the potential for active involvement without multiple steps, which could be frustrating. A therapist would most likely want to avoid "messy" art media such as clay, as clients may be squeamish about getting dirty and may be distracted from the actual task by the material.

All levels of clients benefit from artistic activities in their individual ways. With preparation and planning you can ensure that it is a positive experience for all.

Chapter 6

Therapeutic Art Projects

In this chapter you will find treatment plans using a variety of media for a variety of populations. They are broken down into Collages, Painting and Drawing, Guided Stories, and Miscellaneous. Each plan includes a recommended group size and functioning level, approximate time needed to complete the plan, and the goal or purpose of the process. There will be a list of required or optional materials for the process followed by a step-by-step guide to running the group. I must stress, however, that your own comfort and skill level needs to be taken into account when preparing to implement a group process. If you are unfamiliar or uncomfortable in directing a discussion of issues or feelings, then rework the process to eliminate or reduce the amount of processing needed. Knowing your clients' emotional and physical challenges is also crucial. Art is a door opener. Subconsciously or consciously we all express our emotions through art. Be aware that you may be addressing issues with your clients that they may be resistive to or find uncomfortable to deal with in your group. Make sure a level of trust is established in your group environment and among members. Take the time to develop a supportive core to your group and establish rules early on that address confidentiality, mutual respect, and support among members.

You may want to develop a written group creed or set of rules for higher level groups which address confidentiality issues as well as make the members feel as though they are a part of something unique and special. This "creed" or list of rules can be posted in your art room or handed to new members when they join your group. I have included a sample of a Group Creed I have used (Figure 1), but you may want to draft your own with your group members to address their own unique needs and wishes.

You can further show your respect for the artists by asking them, during the group discussion portion of the project, if they would like to share and talk about their work with the others. Make sure you get the artist's permission to display work and encourage them to take ownership of it by signing and titling the piece, when appropriate. Encourage supportive comments from other participants when showing each member's work. Ask them questions about the feeling of the piece, about the success of the image to create an emotion. Develop an artistic and sensitive eye among the group members so they can further develop their skills and enjoyment during the art making process.

> Explorer's Art Group Creed
>
> As a member of the Explorer's Art Group I agree to treat other members with Respect and Dignity. I will respect the safety and confidentiality of the group members by not discussing with others sensitive issues that may be brought up during our group meeting. I will support the other artists by encouraging their artistic endeavors and sharing my own talents and thoughts during the group time.

Figure 1. Art Group Creed

Collages

I have often underestimated the value of collage work. As an artist myself, I have often thought that an individual's true feelings and emotions cannot be addressed adequately by using images they have not created from scratch. I am reformed. I have seen over and over again that collage work often takes the pressure to perform away from a process and allows real creativity to occur among clients who feel they are not artistically gifted or who are shy or new to a group. It's also a great place to start building a relationship with clients who need one-to-one attention. I have used collage successfully with all populations and although it may take more preparation time, it's worth the effort.

Providing clients with mental illnesses the opportunity to work with images that reflect the "real world" can help open a discussion about perception, as well as issues regarding family, lifestyle, and fear. Clients with dementia or confusion enjoy relating to familiar images and being able to reminisce about better days while in the art process. It provides an occasion for confused or disoriented group members to interact with each other through discussion, and/or shared placement of images on a community piece.

With all populations, collage work takes the initial efforts of image creation away. It allows a client's creativity to show through selection, placement, layering, and the importance an image is given in the piece. It can sometimes help to clearly broadcast an important message from your client, through use of words or images, that they may otherwise have edited out of their design. Some clients are able to disassociate themselves from the emotion they may create because they are "just using the images I could find" when they are actually broadcasting some important thoughts through the arrangement and scheme of their piece.

TIP: Ask a volunteer to go through all your old and donated magazines and cut out large pictures. Divide pictures into categories such as landscapes, holidays, seasons, people, buildings, flowers, etc. and create a file folder for each one. Keep these on hand for your clients who may need inspiration for a painting or drawing, or use them for collage projects! It's great to have them ready when needed, and to dispose of those space-stealing magazine donations.

Sun Images

Size	**4 to 6 medium to low, 10 high**
Functioning	**any level with adaptations**
Time	**preparation time: 20 minutes** **group time: can be done quickly in 30 minutes or can be drawn out into two group sessions**
Purpose	**communication, group interaction, cooperation, fine and gross motor skills**

Mankind has been creating images of the sun since prehistoric times. We find evidence of sun images scratched into cave walls. The sun is part of lore and mythology in all known cultures and is highly regarded as a life giver and provider.

This process uses the theme of the sun as a starting point for creativity. The degree of difficulty and materials used can be adapted for different levels of clients. I will describe a lower level process below (meaning you can do this with moderately confused or early Alzheimer's patients), with some higher level options at the end.

Materials

- black poster board to be cut into 9"x12" sheets as a background piece
- collage images of the sun
- dry glue sticks
- neutral music playing in background

Preparation

Ask a volunteer, or take some time over a few weeks to collect images of the sun. Look in magazine advertisements, travel magazines or brochures, color copy sun images from children's books, or go online to get images. Each image of the sun, plus surrounding environment, should be cropped to a 3"x3" size. You can create a 3"x3" template by cutting out a 3"x3" piece of cardboard, placing it over the sun image, and drawing a line with a pencil around it. Cut on the line. You will need at least twelve images per person, unless you are working as a group on one grid.

Cut black poster board into 9"x12" sheets. Measure 3" increments along the top and side. Draw out a grid of three 3" squares on the top, and four 3" squares down. Draw a heavy line in white pencil (Figure 2).

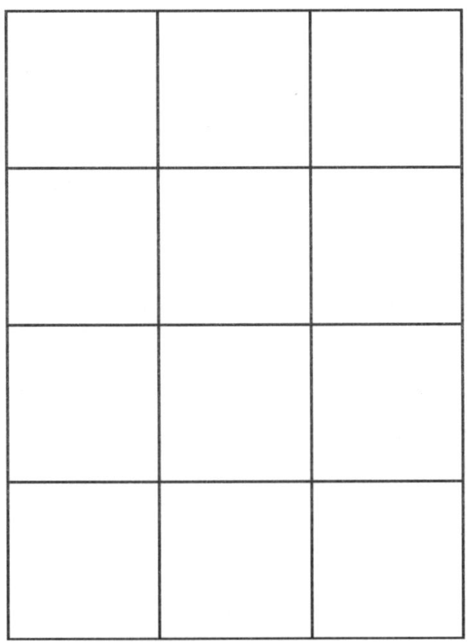

Figure 2. Grid for Sun Images

Project

1. Gather your artists around the table with the sun images laid out within reach.

2. Talk about the significance of the sun and the sun image or symbol. Why might a culture worship the sun? Why do most people just feel better when the sun is shining?

3. Place the black grid-lined boards in front of each person, or use only one for the entire group to work on together.

4. If working as a group, take turns picking out a sun image and gluing it into one of the grid squares on the black poster board. Discuss the image as they work. Why do they like it? Talk about the colors in the image. If working individually, instruct the artists to select images of the sun they like the most and glue them into the grid. If you are working alone and each member of the group needs assistance, ask them to place the suns over the squares and then go around the table and help glue the images into place.

5. When done, you should have an aesthetically interesting collage of sun images that you can display in the day or group room. If you like, you may mount the entire collage on another, larger piece of black poster board to act as a matte. You can also emphasize the grid pattern of the piece by gluing a black ribbon along the lines of the grid or by using colored masking or vinyl tape.

Options

To make this process more challenging for higher level functioning clients, continue with the sun collage theme, but change the materials. Use a fabric background with sun shapes designed by the artists and cut out of different materials, varying the type of fabric, the textures, sizes, and colors. Make sure to include fun and exciting materials like faux fur, metallic fabrics, satin, and burlap. Hot glue the collage to the fabric background and hang sun banners on walls in corridors. Increase the overall size of the project to a 3' x 4' background size and vary the placement and size of sun images. Find some quotes about the sun and, using 3-D fabric paints, write the quote over the piece or across the bottom.

Elements of Life

Size	**6 to 8**
Functioning	**high to medium**
Time	**first session: 20 minutes** **second session: 15 to 20 minutes depending on level of assistance needed**
Purpose	**sensory stimulation, color identification, creativity**

Nature intuitively inspires art. The challenge for most artists is to look at the world around them and to express it on paper, canvas, or film, with all the variance of shades and tones that make it the rich visual feast it is. In the following process clients are asked to look closely at a natural element and to explore the color subtleties present. The use of watercolor paints allows the artist to blend shades and tones easily and spontaneously.

Materials

18"x24" sheets of water color paper; one per person
watercolor paints, brushes, water
thin craft wire
samples or color shades
22"x28" black "railroad" or poster board, one piece per person
hot glue or spray adhesive for mounting materials
nature sound or new age background music

Preparation

As group leader, you need to gather some nature materials before the session. Make sure you have enough to provide an ample number of choices for each client. We also discuss different tones of one true color. Prepare a sample of color shades, or go to a paint store and pick out a paint sample chart, which will show varying degrees of different colors (e.g., various shades of yellow or red).

Each nature element needs to be either 18" or 24" long. Narrow tree or plant branches, such as birch branches, willow branches, stalks from raspberry bushes, with or without leaves, wheat shafts, or even feathers like peacock or eagle work well. (You can buy fake feathers at craft stores for this).

If you have an element that you want to use, but it is not long enough, wire some of the same material together to create a long enough piece.

Project

Session one

1. Begin the group with all the material laid out on tables. Open the group with a discussion of the colors most often found in nature. Talk about the variance of tones in each broad color spectrum. Show an example of how one color can have many "shades" or a "palette" of colors. For example, look at all the different tones of green or black present in your nature materials. Point out how the subtle change of color or tone adds dimension and interest to the object.

2. Ask each person to choose one 18" or 24" length of nature material to use as their inspiration.

3. Turn the watercolor paper so that the chosen material will reach across the entire length of paper. If an artist has chosen an 18" long branch, the paper would be in the 18" wide "portrait" position.

4. Discuss with each artist the subtle tones of color present in the chosen nature material. If a person has chosen a wheat shaft, pick out two color palettes to work with, perhaps a shade of brown and a shade of yellow. Encourage them to create their own color by mixing watercolor paints together.

5. Instruct that on the top **one third** of the paper the artists should perform a "wash" of one of their created color tones. A "wash" is a watery application of color to paper. Wet the paper with clear water to ensure that the application of color goes on smoothly.

6. On the bottom **two thirds** of the paper, instruct the artists to apply a wash of their other color shade. Again wet the paper so that the color applies easily. The two colors should meet and blend or bleed together.

7. Allow the paper to dry. Press them under heavy books to flatten until next session.

Session two

1. Reintroduce the artist to the plan and distribute dried and flattened watercolor paintings and nature objects.

2. Direct the clients to place their nature element at the line where the two colors meet (at the one-third division of the paper). Their branch or material should stretch across the entire length of the paper. Use a 3" to 4" piece of wire and carefully wrap the natural element in two places. Poke the ends of the wire carefully through the watercolor paper. Twist in the back to secure.

3. The entire paper may now be mounted onto black "railroad" or heavy ply poster board using hot glue or spray adhesive on the back of the paper.

4. Discuss the finished projects, title, and display.

The finished project will be a beautiful abstract watercolor painting incorporating and highlighting a piece of nature. The use of watercolor paints rather than acrylic is important here because watercolors offer a more subtle, natural look as opposed to the denser acrylic paint quality.

All the News Fit to Report

Size	**6 to 8**
Functioning	**high to medium**
Time	**30 to 40 minutes**
Purpose	**creativity, discussion, reality orientation, fine and gross motor skills**

The newspaper is an integral part of many people's lives. It keeps us in touch with local and worldwide events, shares opinions, grieves with us over tragedies, and makes us giggle in the funny pages. Still, it is a virtually untapped creative tool for collages! The following project encourages medium to high level clients to look at newspapers, with their headlines, columns, pictures, and maps, as a tool for image making and idea sharing.

In this process we use Masonite boards as a hard background for our collage. Masonite is an inexpensive, pressed fiberboard that is usually used by artists as a base for creation of a paint board canvas. Here we use it for its solid, warp-resistant qualities and its ability to stand up to multiple layers of glue and paper.

Materials

daily newspapers including advertisements, comics; all parts of the paper (Sunday newspapers tend to have more color images, so use them if you can.)
18"x24" Masonite panels, one per person
Mod Podge glue/glazing medium
paint brushes or sponge brushes
plastic gloves

Project

1. Begin the process with a discussion about the news. How many in the group read the newspaper? Ask "Why or Why not?"
2. Let the artists know that they will be working with printed newspapers as an art medium. Ask them to go through the newspapers supplied, and to select pages or sections that have news they feel is interesting or vital to them, sections that have powerful or playful stories or pictures, or anything that they would like to incorporate into a collage. They should include headlines as well as smaller articles. They could think of a theme and collect articles and pictures around that, or just select parts at random.
3. Separate their selections into black and white and color images.
4. Place a Masonite board in front of each artist, along with a brush and a supply of Mod Podge glue/glaze. Artists may choose to wear plastic gloves here if they do not want to get glue on their hands.
5. Instruct artists to tear their selections of newsprint into large, irregular shapes and apply to the Masonite by first brushing the Masonite with the Mod Podge medium, then applying the paper over the glaze, followed by more Mod Podge on top.
6. They should apply most of the black and white print first, making sure to cover the entire board. Overlapping pieces will be necessary and desirable. Don't let the clients get held up with trying to make entire articles or words readable. Remind them that they are using it, as they would paint or markers. Being able to read the article is not necessary; we just want the idea of it.
7. Next, choose three or four pieces of colored newsprint, tear, and place over the black and white in a few areas.
8. When finished, brush the entire surface with a thin layer of the glaze.
9. When all are done, discuss the finished projects.

Possible discussion questions:

- Does the piece have a theme?
- Did you select a series of articles or pictures with certain significance to you?
- When you look at other pieces what do you think?
- Do the colors and the headlines indicate a theme or a title to you?

End the group with a discussion about the news and our need to see and hear important news, as well as good news.

Allow boards to dry and display with titles.

Looks like a Celebration!

Size	**4 to 6 low, 8 medium and high**
Functioning	**any levels with adaptations**
Time	**20 to 35 minutes**
Purpose	**playfulness and creativity, reminiscence, gross motor skills, group socialization**

Do you remember the joy and spontaneity you had when you were a kid while opening gifts — the sheer thrill of ripping paper and shredding tissue, casting ribbons aside and wearing bows on your head.

The following process encourages a sense of play with all level of clients in a reminiscent attitude toward the holiday season. You may have to part with some of your own used gift wrap stash for this splashy, spontaneous, and fun collage process.

Materials

new or used wrapping paper in a variety of sizes
metallic ribbons cut into two to three foot pieces
solid glue stick
black railroad board (6 ply medium weight) 22"x28" cut in half (one half board per person)
spray glue
glitter
optional: clear contact paper, metallic art papers

Preparation

Before group begins, have black poster board and a glue stick at each persons work area. Have all the other materials in middle of the table in a big, messy pile. (It's just more fun that way.)

Project

1. When members are seated, discuss childhood gift opening traditions. Ask questions such as, “Do you remember ripping through wrapping paper with abandon? Can you remember what the floor looked like at home after unwrapping gifts? Were there ribbons and wrapping remnants lying all over the house?”
2. Ask: “What if you could recreate the joy that was felt then in a collage?”
3. Shuffle through the materials on the table, instruct the artists to randomly select papers, rip them up into any size pieces, and glue them on to the board. Tell them they are trying to recreate the spontaneity and thrill that a child has during gift opening. They shouldn’t plan too much, but select colors and patterns that appeal to them. They could even just throw the papers up in the air and glue them in place if they wanted!
4. Ribbons can be added to enhance the 3-D effect of the collage by layering them between wrapping pieces and gluing them in place. If they would like more shine to their piece, they may add some glitter by lightly spraying glue over the desired area and sprinkling glitter onto it. Shake off the excess.
5. When all the pieces are glued down, you may opt to cover the entire piece with clear contact paper to keep everything in place and to seal it. I prefer leaving it well glued, but uncovered, since the contact paper can somewhat flatten colors and detract from the piece.
6. Show each piece and ask the artist to give it a title.

Display

To enhance and explain the concept of this project, you could type up the stories the artists told about remembered gift openings and display this as well (with their permission, of course).

All in all, this is a fun and lighthearted process that invites all cognitive and physical functioning clients to participate. The discussion and reminiscence is very important to the process and should be encouraged.

If working with clients who have Alzheimer's, the "scattered" and unorganized feel of this process might be more difficult for them. I suggest using one piece of poster board to do a group project on, and focus mostly on the reminiscence, gross and fine motor skills, and the ability to follow directions. You may take more time in looking at the patterns on the wrapping paper and the shimmer of the ribbons. Plan ahead and ask family members to bring in old pictures of family gift opening times or parties to add a special touch to the project.

Bits of Africa

Size	**6 to 8**
Functioning	**medium to high; low with adaptations**
Time	**35 minutes**
Purpose	**cultural appreciation, discussion, fine and gross motor skills, creativity, self-expression**

The following process celebrates both the African culture and the beauty of nature. We will combine the use of wildlife patterned paper with a bit of the Swahili language to bring forth a vibrant collage that is not only visually but also mentally stimulating. It can be done with all cognitive levels of clients, with varying degrees of assistance.

Materials

wildlife patterned paper (available at Sax Arts and Crafts under "Amazing Animal Paper" #415-4225; call 1-800-558-6696)
solid glue sticks
black poster board or railroad board, to be used as a background piece, cut into 11"x14" sheets (one per person)
photographs of Africa to display
Swahili words (see end of project) enlarged and cut out
sample of project without Swahili words on it
African music to play in background

Preparation

Cut the wildlife print paper into different shapes and sizes. Determine what print pattern you want for each shape and cut them. Shapes may be different sizes, but should remain constant with the print paper.

For example, all the leopard paper will be cut into circles of various sizes, all the zebra paper will be cut into squares of various sizes, etc.

Enlarge the Swahili words found at the end of this project and cut them out. Words should be no larger than what can fit on an 8.5"x11" paper. Alternatively, you could use a wide-tipped black marker and cursively write the words over the collage.

You can also retype the words on your computer and print them onto clear adhesive paper. Then, simply stick the whole sheet over the collage (www.decalpaper.com has the clear adhesive paper, but you should also be able to find it at your local office supply store).

Project

1. Let the participants know that the project they are working on today will be in celebration of Africa and the beauty of the country. Begin by showing photographs of Africa and talking about the country and culture.
2. Lay out all the patterned papers within reach of the clients and distribute the black poster board background sheets.
3. Discuss the beauty of nature, and of the patterns they see before them. Can they identify the animal that inspired the pattern?
4. Ask, "If you had to compare yourself to one of the animals represented, which one would you choose?" "Why?"
5. Using the papers before them, they are to create a collage of wildlife prints to fill the surface of their black poster board. (Show a sample)
6. They should layer their papers, using the different shapes, colors, and sizes to create patterns. Encourage them not to use all of one type of animal, although they may start off with the animal they feel the most affinity with.
7. As they begin to move their collage materials around, bring out glue sticks and assist with gluing as necessary. The process should take about 20 to 30 minutes.

8. When complete, bring out your enlarged Swahili words. Discuss the meanings of the words. Try saying the words together. (Make a copy of the words and meanings for them to take with them). Ask each person to choose a word they find most meaningful and to apply it over the top of their collage as an accent.

Display

When complete, display the pieces together with a note on the process of the session.

NOTE: For lower level clients, use smaller background paper and concentrate on animal pattern identification, following directions, and fine and gross motor skills. Be prepared to do all the gluing for your clients as necessary.

The following Swahili words were found on the below listed web site. Please visit this site to add more words to you list if you desire.

The Kamusi Project Internet Living Swahili Dictionary
http://www.yale.edu/swahili/

love - ashiki
faith - dini
family - ahali
courage - uhodari
hope - matarajio
dream - njozi
freedom from care - mteremo
good day - jambo

Fantasy Landscapes

Size	**6 to 8**
Functioning	**medium to high, lower with adaptations**
Time	**preparation: 30 to 40 minutes** **group time: 35 to 40 minutes**
Purpose	**creativity, art instruction, abstract thinking**

The following project challenges medium to high level clients to see and create a world in a different way. Using photocopied or scanned close-ups of familiar materials, group members are excited to explore the textural possibilities in this fun and easy plan. Group members will also get a chance to discuss basic landscape composition and to apply what they know to this collage process.

Materials

scanned or photocopied textural images
dry glue sticks
scissors
9"x12" black construction paper
landscape photographs as inspiration (can be found in magazines such as *National Geographic*)
optional: colored pencils

Preparation

Photocopy (or scan on your computer) a variety of texturally different and unusual items: a string of lights (bunched up on copier), folds in fabric, a pile of nails or screws, leaves, feathers, etc. Make at least ten copies of each textured pattern and cut away from the background so clients only see a close-up of the texture. See the example towel texture (Figure 3).

Project

1. Begin the group with a discussion of landscapes. Looking at a sample, talk about the different elements in a landscape. There are usually three basic divisions. The bottom of the photo might contain water, or grasses. The middle might contain mountains or buildings, and the top most likely highlights the sky — day or nighttime.

2. Invite your group to construct a landscape using unusual textures from familiar sources. Exhibit the scans or photocopies you have prepared. Can they guess what the item you have featured is? Ask them to look closely at each texture. Can they relate the lines or the feel of that texture to some landscape element you discussed? For example, do the folds in the fabric look like sand dunes or water?

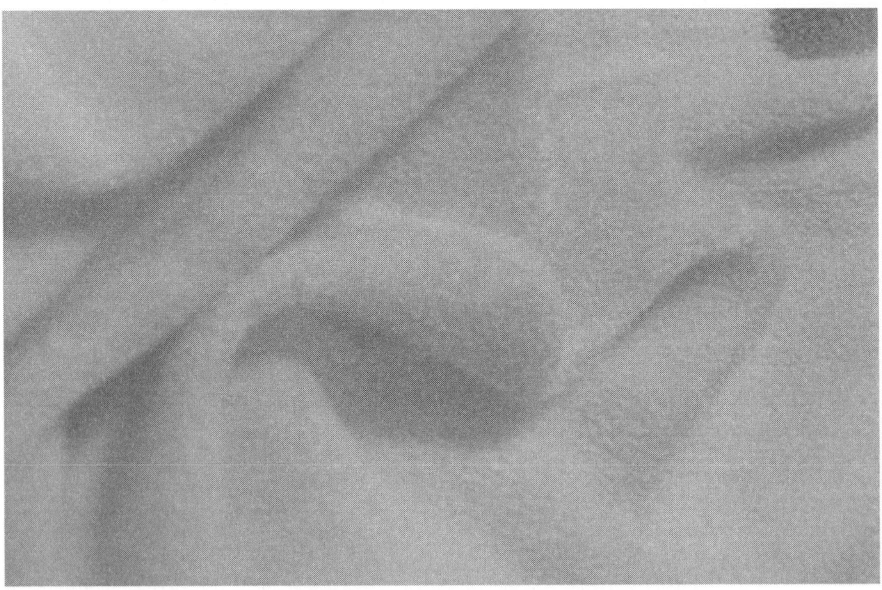

Figure 3. Towel Texture Sample

3. With each artist armed with several sheets of each texture and the black construction paper, challenge them to play with the composition and create their own fantasy landscapes. They may use scissors to trim down or otherwise shape the textural images.

4. NOTE: It's great if you were able to scan or copy the textures in color. If not, feel free to allow the clients to lightly go over

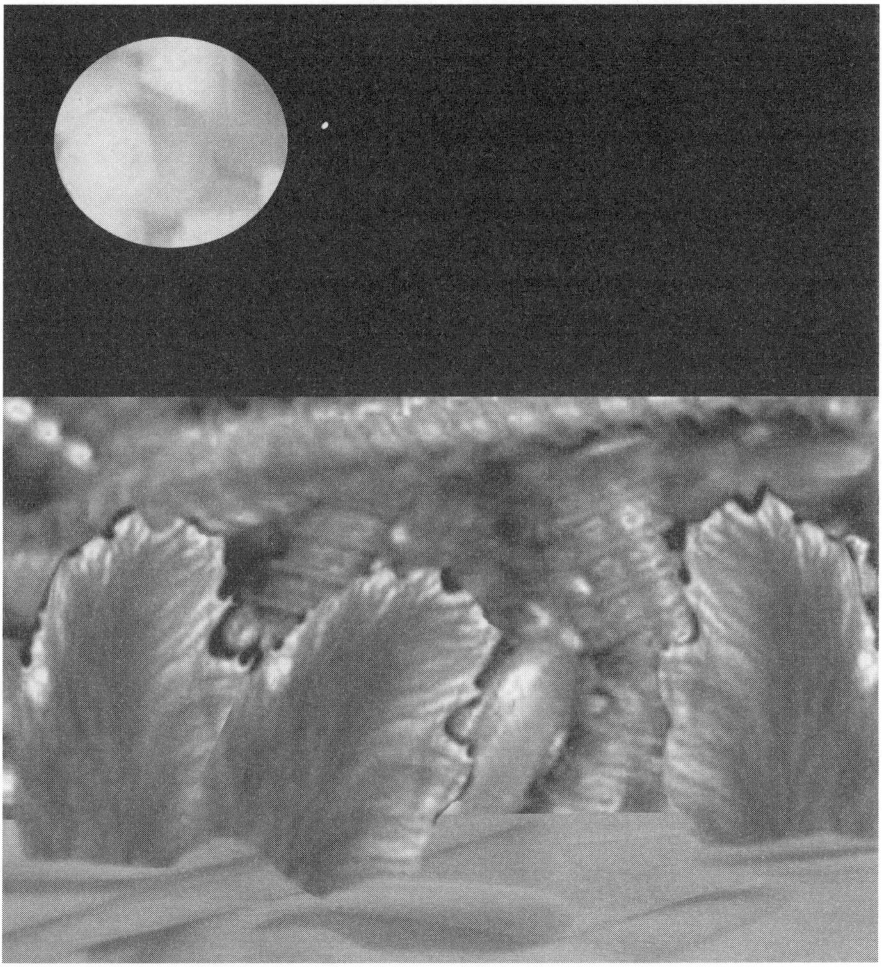

Figure 4. Fantasy Landscape

different elements with colored pencils to create a hand colored effect.

5. Encourage the repeated use and layering of the same texture to create a series of hills or grasses, for example. Remind them that elements may be turned and trimmed to achieve the effect they may want.

6. When the composition is complete, trim off or crop excess background paper to focus the piece.

7. When all members are done, ask each artist to name his or her creation. Then matte and display, with permission.

Display

See Figure 4 for a sample of a finished landscape using holiday lights, nails, feathers, and folded material images.

NOTE: The leftover texture images may be used with lower level clients as part of a sensory stimulation group. Ask them to identify the source of the image, and then introduce them to the original item. For example, show the clients a close-up of the feathers and then bring out actual feathers! You may also want to challenge them by showing the finished landscapes from your art group. Can they dissect the pictures and match items you bring along with the items in the art piece?

Running Circles

Size	**6 to 8**
Functioning	**any level with adaptations**
Time	**20 to 30 minutes**
Purpose	**fine motor skills, sensory stimulation, art appreciation, creativity, discussion**

Roy Lichtenstein was a well-known pop artist of the 1960s. His best known works, such as *I...I'm Sorry* (1965 to 1966) resemble large comic book illustrations. His graphic works, in all their complexity, highlight the use of dots or colored circles to create shape, light, and shadow. Lichtenstein's work was the inspiration for the following art project that can be implemented to suit low level clients as well as higher level clients. (See the end of the project for low-level adaptations.)

This process does require some preparation work, so plan ahead and solicit volunteers to help if you can.

Materials

- colored paper: metallic, glossy, patterned, and flat color (variety of fabrics for low-level adaptations)
- scissors
- dry glue sticks (liquid glue and/or hot glue for adaptations)
- white pencils
- black poster board 11"x14" sheets — one per person
- samples of Lichtenstein's work to show (look for *I...I'm Sorry* and *Vicki* online)
- 8"x10" close-up images of flowers or landscapes (go to www.webshots.com to check out their wide variety of images you can download and use for this project.)

Preparation

Cut the colored and patterned papers into ½" or 1" circles (whichever will work best with your photos and clients).

Project

1. Begin the group with a discussion of Lichtenstein's work. Talk about how an image can be created by gathering dots of color together to create shadow, form, and detail. Talk about how a variety of tones and shades put together can create shape.
2. Ask artists to choose a photograph that they will deconstruct down to its "dots" components. Talk about taking a realistic image and turning it into a more abstract representation of itself.
3. Pass out black poster board, glue sticks, and precut circles.
4. Depending on the level of your group, they may choose to use the image for inspiration and work from scratch on the black poster board, or they may choose to glue the photo onto the poster board and overlay the entire image with the colored dots. Either way, their creation should resemble an abstract version of the original photograph. (See Figure 5.) NOTE: For very high level groups, artists may choose to create a design of their own invention using the dots. They may sketch the image out on the poster board in white pencil and fill in with dots.
5. When complete, title the work and display.

Adaptations

- For lower level groups, make the circles larger (3" to 4") and include some fabric and other textural varieties. Using a large 22"x24" sheet of poster board, sketch out a large, open flower design and take turns filling in the design with colored circles. Circles can overlay one another and can be a mix of fabric and paper. (Use liquid glue or assist with hot glue for fabrics.)

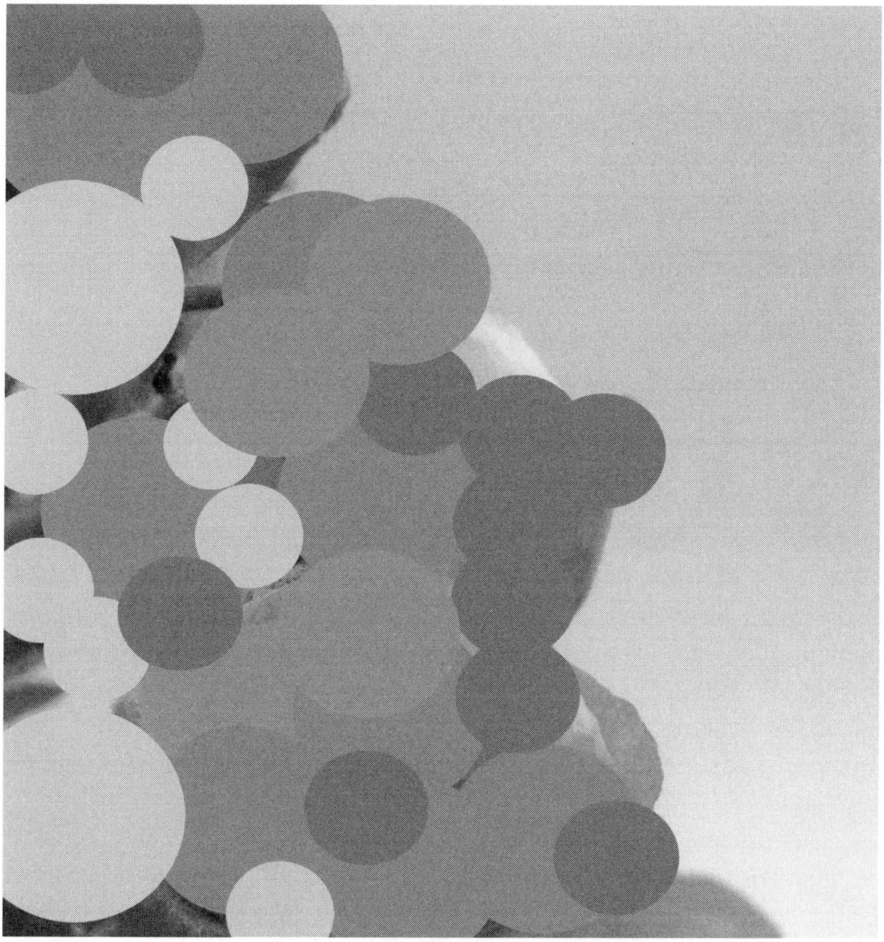

Figure 5. Running Circles

Watery Blooms

Size	**6 to 8**
Functioning	**medium to high**
Time	**first session: 20 to 30 minutes** **second session: 20 minutes**
Purpose	**concrete and abstract thinking, fine motor skills, creativity, art instruction**

While working on a computer art program one day, I realized that high-tech art software offers some ideas that can be done in low-tech ways. Case in point: photo manipulation programs. Programs like Adobe Photoshop often provide options for turning parts of your original photography into watercolor paintings, ink drawings, or even embossed images! With this in mind, I thought it might be fun to work with glossy magazine images and beautiful, flowing paints to create the same mixture of concrete image and abstract background available through the computer.

This process is best done with medium to high level clients, but can be done with lower level clients as well with hand-over-hand assistance. I also suggest completing it in two sessions to give the background artwork ample time to dry.

For this particular technique, I use vibrant, high intensity India inks instead of watercolor paints to give the final image more impact.

Materials

- medium to large magazine pictures of flowers, cut away from surrounding images
- watercolor paper (full sheet is usually 22"x30")
- colored inks (such as Dr. Martin's Bombay India Inks)
- spray bottles with water

spray adhesive and/or dry glue sticks
3-D paints or black permanent markers
broad tipped watercolor brushes
table coverings
paper toweling
black display or poster board for mounting

Project

Session one

1. Begin the group by discussing the use of colored India inks. On a small piece of wet watercolor paper, demonstrate how inks can be applied using the eyedropper, and show how colors can be encouraged to bleed together with the use of additional water and brushes. Talk about the "watery" effect the application creates. NOTE: Too many colors mixed together will give you a muddy look. Be selective with color choices.

2. Discuss how they will use this abstract art technique to compliment and enhance a flower image of their choice.

3. Distribute flower images (each artist chooses one) and discuss the primary colors of each image. These primary colors will determine which inks they should use.

4. Placing the flower images aside, pass out full sheets of watercolor paper that have been wetted either by submersion in a tray of water or by spraying with water.

5. Sharing the inks, the artists may now apply the colors needed, spraying or brushing slightly to create the wet, moving color look desired. (The less actual brush application used, the better the final image will be.)

6. When all colors have been applied, you may soak up some of the excess water by carefully laying paper toweling gently over image. Do not rub or pat down.

7. Allow all paintings to dry thoroughly. Weight papers down with heavy books to flatten dry paintings.

Session two

1. Place the original flower picture and painting in front of the artist.
2. Looking at the ink painting, ask the artist to place the picture on the paper, either in the center, or in an especially vibrant area of the painting.
3. Using spray adhesive or dry glue sticks, attach the picture to the painting.
4. Areas of the painting can be highlighted or accented if desired using 3-D paints or markers.
5. Crop the painting as desired, and mount onto black poster or display board.

Notes

- Save cropped paper to use in other collage techniques, or to create small gift tags or cards in the future. The final project will be an incorporation of traditional original art and modern imagery. Mounted on black, they should create a vibrant and interesting visual for the artists and their supporters.
- India ink is permanent ink. Latex gloves or painting smocks might be appropriate for your clients.

Fine Art Deconstruction

Size	**6 to 8**
Functioning	**high to medium; low with adaptations**
Time	**preparation: one hour**
	group time: 30 to 40 minutes
Purpose:	**abstract thinking, discussion, fine motor skills, creativity**

This process utilizes fine art reproductions, a selected color theme, and collage techniques to create design and visual interest without the fear of creating something that might fail or be aesthetically unsatisfying. The use of fine art as a collage material will give the final image a rich, dramatic look not available through use of flat colored paper.

Materials

- art reproductions with selected main colors
- glue sticks
- black poster board cut into 12"x16" sheets
- large white poster boards in 16"x20" sheets
- 4"x4" viewfinder that you make (see end of project)
- scissors
- soft music

Preparation

The main challenge in this process is in the preparation. Go to some art history books or other good quality books with large illustrations (finely illustrated fairy tale books are also good) and find some with large blocks of colors. Select rich warm tones for the most dramatic final pieces. You can also find image sources by going to the web sites www.nowsurrealgalleries.co.uk/artist, www.artmagick.com, or www.allposters.com and search through the artwork there.

To use that artwork, right click with your mouse over artwork that has the right color schemes and "copy" then "paste" the image in a blank Word document, enlarge, and print. Although the image might be grainy, that is all right, you are really only using it for the colors, not the images.

Once you have color-printed or machine copied the images you have found in books or on the Internet, use your viewfinder to isolate areas of the image that have interesting color and shapes and outline in pen. Cut out the blocks and put aside for group. NOTE: high and medium level clients could do this step.

Cut the 4"x4" image in half.

Before the group begins you should have at least ten blocks of each color for each client.

Project

1. To begin the group, discuss the different kinds of art available, (fine art, classical, abstract, illustrations) and show whole image samples of each. Next talk about color. Discuss the various shades and tones of colors. Talk about how certain colors make us feel different emotions.

2. Next, challenge your artists to use color samples of published artwork to create a new and interesting image.

3. Place the black poster board in front of each artist as their background piece. Pass out glue sticks. Place the collage materials out on the table in like-color piles.

4. Allow the artists to look at the color blocks. Discuss how you got the blocks and see if they can identify any images in them. Each artist will select one set to work with (staying within a color scheme).

5. With soft music playing in the background, invite the clients to simply use the collage materials to create an image on the black background. They may use the blocks in a circle, line them up,

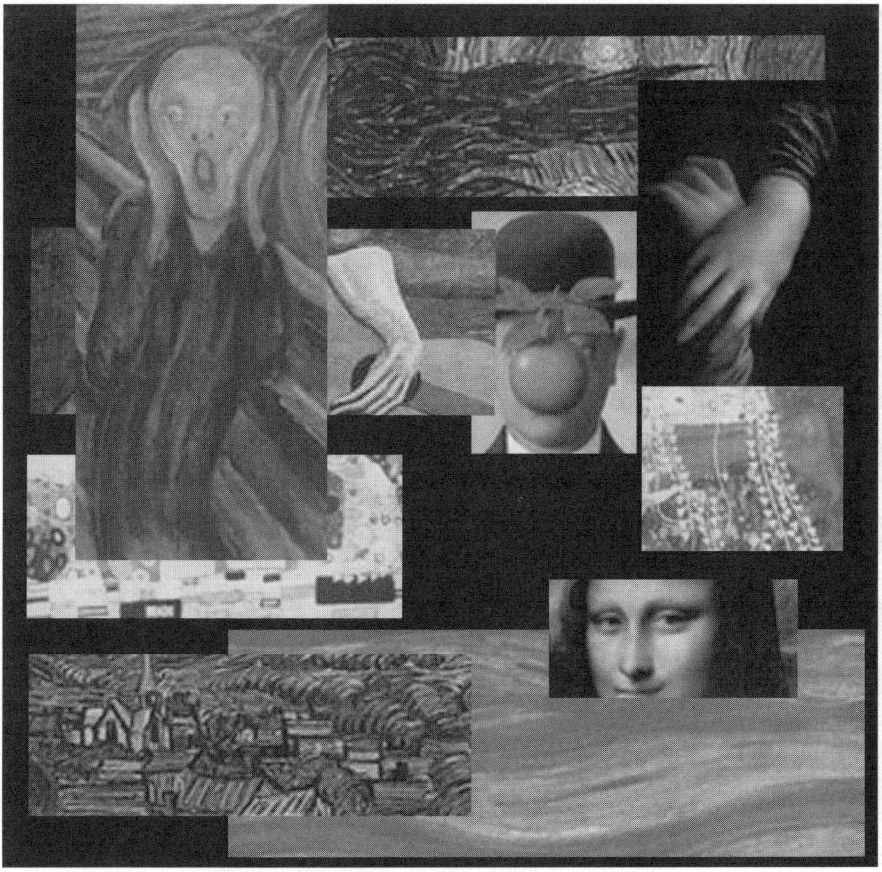

Figure 6. Fine Art Deconstruction 1

or overlap them. Anything goes! (You might want to make a smaller sample to help them get the idea.) They should cover as much of the black paper as possible.

6. Allow 20 minutes or so to complete the project. Since this is a non-threatening form of art, clients may enjoy talking quietly to one another, sharing collage materials, discussing the art reproductions, etc.

7. When complete, mount each black poster board to the larger white board, which will act as a matte. Ask each participant to show their final project to the other members. Discuss the use of

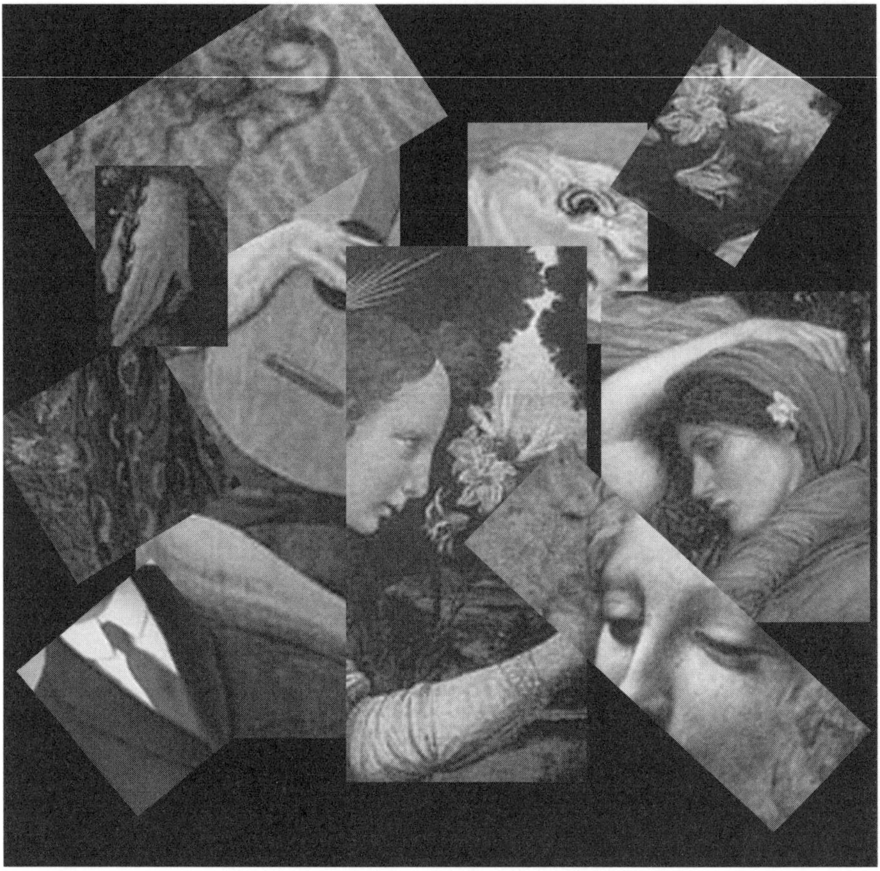

Figure 7. Fine Art Deconstruction 2

abstract color forms derived from fine art as collage materials. See Figure 6 and Figure 7 for a sample of what the final images might look like.

Options

1. If you don't have a color printer and Internet access you may (or ask a volunteer to) search through fashion or women's magazines for advertisements which feature shades of one color or large areas of one color that you can cut out. For example, many

perfume or jewelry advertisements feature their product in a blue light, or against a red velvet background.

2. Try using different faces from art, or eyes, or hands… anything you can imagine as a theme, or allow clients to work from all color schemes.

3. For lower level groups, leave the images in 4"x4" blocks and reduce the paper size to 12"x12". Ask clients to do a collage using all shades of one color and challenge them to find the colors in a larger pile of images.

Making a viewfinder: Take a piece of poster board and cut it into a 6"x6" square. Cut a 4"x4" hole in the middle. Move the viewfinder over artwork or advertisements to isolate beautiful colors and abstract forms.

Celebrating the Colors of Mexico

Size	**6 to 8**
Functioning	**medium to high; low with adaptations**
Time	**30 to 40 minutes**
Purpose	**art education, cultural exploration, fine motor skills, self-expression**

This process explores the traditional colors and history of Mexican folk art. It is meant to be a creative way to celebrate and learn about the culture. The traditional colors of Mexico are beautiful and vibrant. When used together, they naturally create an exciting and visually interesting art piece.

Materials

- extra bright colored construction paper or Origami paper cut into 4"x4" pieces
- scissors
- solid glue sticks
- bright yellow colored poster board, cut into strips 4"x 22", one piece per person (to be used as a background piece)
- samples of traditional Mexican folk art and designs
- black markers for outlining patterns
- Mexican music in background

Project

1. Show samples of traditional Mexican art and designs. (You can look up Mexican art, Aztec art, or Mayan art online to find some sources.) Discuss the use of nature as inspiration for many of the designs (sun patterns, nature object and animal motifs).

2. Pass out the bright yellow background paper, and place the colored square paper within reach on the table.
3. Listening to the Mexican music, ask the artists to draw and cut designs out of the colored paper. Each design should utilize as much of the 4"x4" square as possible. (Have a sample for viewing so they get the idea of what the finished project could look like). Use the Mexican artwork samples as inspiration. Discuss using sun, animal, and human images as symbols in their artwork.
4. As they cut out each design, they may lay it out on the yellow background paper to create a band pattern, applying each design directly next to the previous piece. Artists may repeat the same form over and over, or may utilize many different colors and forms to create their piece (Figure 8).
5. Once they have filled the 22" band (cut the band shorter if necessary), glue all the pieces down onto the band.
6. Display bands together with an explanation of the inspiration for the group.

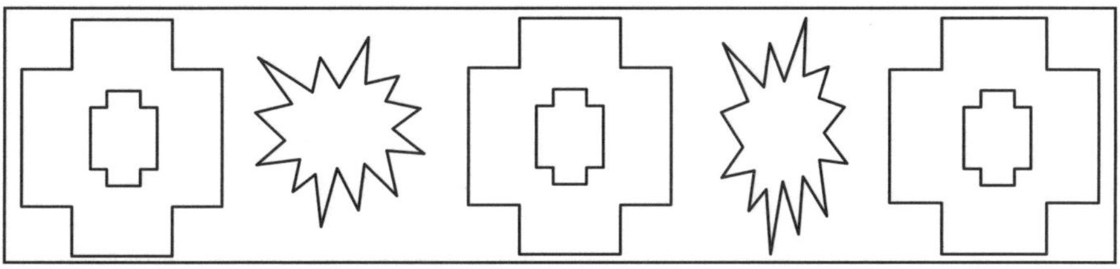

Figure 8. Celebrating the Colors of Mexico

Adaptations

For lower level clients, pre-cut traditional Mexican shapes out of the colored paper squares, and focus the group on following directions and color identification. All client levels can appreciate the Mexican influence by listening to the music and by utilizing the colorful shapes to create a vibrant pattern.

Tissue Paper Painting

Size	**6 to 8**
Functioning	**high**
Time	**preparation: 20 minutes** **group time: 30 to 40 minutes (may take more than one session)**
Purpose	**art education, creativity, fine motor skills, following directions, abstract thinking**

The following project uses non-threatening materials and magazine photographs to teach clients how to look at the world around them as bits of color and shapes and to enjoy the act of art creation.

This project requires some fine motor skills and patience. It can even be done with clients with mild visual deficits. If they can see blocks of colors, they can do this process. It's not about details; it's about blurring the lines and definitions of what they see.

By applying the mosaic of tissue paper directly on top of the original piece (as described below), the client can see the transformation from concrete or "realistic" art to abstract.

Materials

craft tissue paper in a variety of colors
dry glue sticks
magazine photos
Mod Podge glue/glaze
9"x12" cut sheets of black matte board
clear adhesive tape

Preparation

1. Tear sheets of tissue paper into small pieces (approximately 2"x2") and keep separated by color.

2. Look through magazines such as *National Geographic*, gardening magazines, or travel magazines and cut out large (8"x11" preferably), close-up pictures of flowers, broad landscapes, or simple nature scenes. The larger, clearer, and simpler the picture is, the better.

Project

1. Place the colored tissue paper on the tables within reach of the artists. Let them know that they will be creating an abstract piece of art based on a magazine picture they choose. They will be using the colored tissue paper in a mosaic fashion to "paint" their image.

2. Lay magazine pictures out on the table. Ask each person to choose one that he or she likes. Tape the edges of the magazine photo down onto the table in front of them to avoid having it slip and move while working.

3. Ask them to identify the primary colors they notice in the photographs.

4. Artists should take the colored tissue paper they need, based on the identified colors, and pile some near their work area.

5. Using the dry glue stick, they are to apply glue to a small area on the magazine photo, select colored tissue that matches it, and apply the tissue directly onto the photo. They should tear the tissue paper into smaller pieces as needed and overlap colors or pieces to build interest and fill in the shapes. (Demonstrating this in front of the group will help get them on the right track.)

6. They should continue to glue up small areas of the picture and cover with tissue until the whole picture is covered. (This may take more than one session.)

7. Cover your 9"x12" matte board with Mod Podge and adhere the completed piece onto it. Brush Mod Podge over the entire piece to seal and lay down any remaining loose edges.

The resulting pieces should be a loose and abstract mosaic of tissue. Whether it still looks like the original picture is not important. The process of seeing the particles that make up an image, and using that as an inspiration is the most important thing.

The true success of this project lies in finding the most appropriate magazine pictures. I have found the easiest pictures are close-ups of flower blossoms. The large petals and contrast of blossom color to green leaf color makes this project go quickly and easily. If your clients are more advanced, or for future projects, challenge them to use this technique with large portrait pictures or other landscapes. Another way to approach the same process is to just cover one half or a third of the photo image with tissue and leave the rest untouched. This provides a type of multimedia collage look that can be very dramatic and visually interesting.

Geological Art

Size	**6 to 8**
Functioning	**any level with adaptations**
Time	**25 minutes**
Purpose	**education, creativity, fine and gross motor skills, discussion**

The inspiration for this project is the beauty of sedimentary rock layers. Over billions of years the earth has been a work in process. Geologists can see evidence of past animals, weather, and plant life as they dig down through the earth and study the layers. Showing your clients some of these images (go online and search under sedimentary rocks) will inspire them to tear through the materials provided to create an earthy and aesthetically interesting ripped paper collage.

The following project uses colored charcoal or pastel drawing paper as the media for this multidimensional torn paper collage. The textural qualities of this 25 lb. weight paper, along with its nice edge when ripped, make it a good alternative for colored construction paper, and gives this process a more adult feel.

Materials

drawing paper of various colors 19"x25" sheets (plan for at least four sheets per person)
black railroad board (22"x28") in 6-ply for mounting
dry glue sticks or double sided tape
photos of sedimentary rocks
music

Project

1. Begin the group with a discussion of the layers of the earth. Show pictures of sedimentary rocks with their beautiful layers of color.

2. Taking inspiration from those layers of earth, invite the artists to choose four different colors of paper to create their own layered art.

3. Begin by crinkling up all the sheets of paper into balls and then flattening out again. This gives the sheets an increased dimensional and textural quality that's beneficial for this process.

4. Ask artists to select one color for their background piece. That piece should remain intact, and can be dry glued to the middle of the black railroad board.

5. Taking a second sheet of a different color, instruct artists to pinch the paper in spots and tear holes in it. The torn paper parts can be ripped into different abstract shapes. They could out tear one large section or several smaller holes in the paper. However, the paper itself should remain in one piece. Place that layer over the background layer.

6. Repeat the above process with the remaining two colors of paper. Layering the sheets, the clients will see only parts of the layer beneath peeking through. As they work, they may decide to tear more from lower layers so that other colors are more visible.

7. When satisfied, dry glue all layers together onto the railroad board background.

The final piece should be a peek-a-boo of colors and textures reminiscent of a sedimentary rock formation. (See Figure 9.)

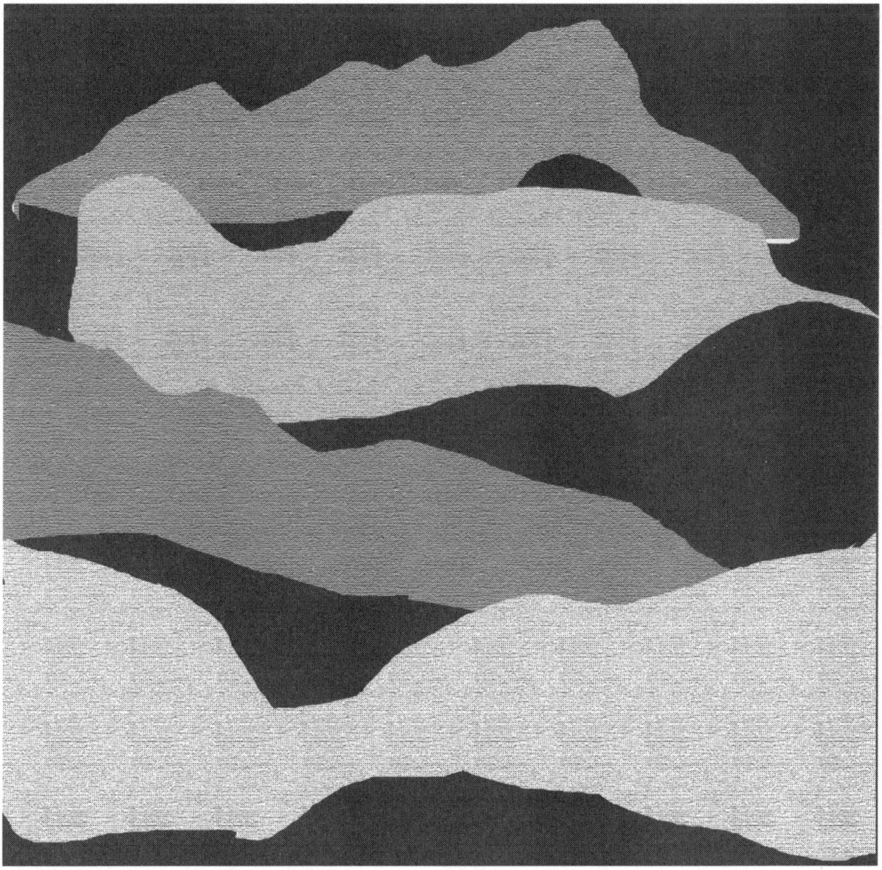

Figure 9. Geological Art

Adaptation

This process can be done with lower level clients by simply tearing the colored paper into strips and asking them to layer them onto the base color paper. The focus here would be discussion, group interaction, fine motor skills, and following directions.

Painting/Drawing

Painting groups hold a few more challenges than collage plans. There are more technical points involved, and they can be a bit too messy or complicated for more confused clients. However, the act of brushing paint onto a surface can be very soothing for all populations. With supervision (and even hand-over-hand assistance), creating large, abstract murals with even your lowest level clients can be achievable and beneficial. One must be aware of pitfalls like muddying colors. (When too many colors are blended together you most often end up with brown!) You must also make sure you have the right tools and plenty of preparation and clean up time. Buy quality brushes. Less expensive brushes inevitably shed hairs onto the work and your clients will spend their time attempting to pick them out for the duration of the group. Make sure you have ample water for cleaning brushes between color applications and plenty of paper toweling for wiping up spills and wiping excess paint off brushes. Painting smocks or aprons may be appropriate for these projects.

Light into Darkness

Size	**6 to 8**
Functioning	**high to medium**
Time	**30 to 40 minutes**
Purpose	**discussion, self-expression, creativity, gross motor skills**

This group combines professional quality materials and a theme of "bringing light into the darkness." Artists are asked to paint over a black background with brighter colors as an example of how even the darkest situations can be changed to something brighter.

We use large canvas panels, which are sized, primed, and ready to go for this process. They are available at most arts and craft supply stores. I choose to use this canvas to offer the artists a feeling of professionalism, to provide a good foundation for the acrylic paints we will be using, and to create a finished look to our final project without the trouble of mattéing the work later.

Materials

large sponge brushes for background color application
acrylic paints, all colors dispensed in individual palettes or paint cups
canvas panels 11"x14"
a variety of sizes of soft, round paintbrushes, at least one 1" brush per person
water buckets
paper toweling
clear tape
inspirational photographs
3"x3" viewfinders

table coverings
background music (light classical or new age)

Preparation

1. Collect some large, bright, and colorful close-up images of flowers. You should be able to find these in gardening magazines, old flower calendars, old greeting cards, or even online. (Search under "hi res flower images" then use a color printer to print them out for the group.)

2. Create viewfinders to help narrow the artist's focus on one area of color and shape. Cut a 3"x3" square in the middle of an 8"x11" piece of paper. The artist will slide the viewfinder over images to select areas of interest.

3. Prepare the 11"x14" canvases. Using a large sponge brush, coat each canvas with a solid application of black paint. Do this a day or two ahead of group time so the paint is dry. (Enlist some resident volunteers to help!) This is done to create a dark background for the vibrant paint colors and to create a more finished look to the piece when through. Using acrylic paints on top of the black background will give the top colors more depth, show off the textures of brush strokes and shapes, and automatically fill in the unused areas of the canvas. This also works with our theme of "bringing light into the darkness" by allowing the bright top colors to overcome the original pitch of the canvas.

4. Before the artists arrive, have tables covered, canvases and paints dispensed, water containers, brushes, and paper toweling at each place. Have music playing in background and, if possible, have a small canvas prepared for you to demonstrate on. Have flower images out in middle of work surface, with viewfinders at each client's work area.

Project

1. When all members have come into the room, begin a discussion about feeling blue or depressed. Have they ever felt like there was no "light at the end of the tunnel?" What has helped them get through this period? Talk about how some people feel that even when things look their darkest, something wonderful will happen and turn the whole situation around. For example, a person may wake up grumpy and irritable. Then a friendly smile or a nice compliment from someone else may just turn that whole mood around! Talk about how they will be illustrating that point by bringing a beautiful image to a once dark and bleak canvas.

2. Ask members to look through the photographs and to select an image they find appealing. They may choose one because of the colors, shapes, or just the way the image makes them feel.

3. Using the viewfinders, ask them to isolate one area of the image to use as inspiration for their acrylic paintings. Tape the viewfinders in place over the original picture.

4. Demonstrate, if possible, how they will be "bringing light into the darkness" by using vibrant colors over the black canvases. Using a heavy application of paint, illustrate how texture and line, against the black background, can create an exciting effect. By showing the group members a quick example, they will feel less pressure to "re-create" their images and will be able to explore the use of paints on the black canvas more freely.

5. Reinforce the idea that they are to "work big" and not be afraid to use broad strokes and bright colors. They may also elaborate on the design they see through their viewfinders. Encourage them to let their imaginations flow and to create with joy and lack of censorship.

6. Allow the group to work for 20 minutes.

7. When complete, clear tables of extraneous paints, toweling, and papers. One by one ask members to show their work if they like and discuss the process.
8. Display canvases in a group.

If possible, surprise your artists with real flowers to take back to their rooms at the end of the group! This will give them a conversation starter with peers and staff and will remind them of their worth in your group.

Courage

Size	**8 to 10**
Functioning	**high to medium**
Time	**30 minutes**
Purpose	**discussion, motivation, abstract thinking**

Living in an institutional setting can be a scary experience. Being away from family and friends, in limited control of comings and goings, and the uncertainty of health issues, can create an environment of anxiety and fear. It's good to remind ourselves occasionally that we have the ability to overcome and to triumph no matter what the odds.

The following project talks about courage with high to medium level cognitive functioning clients and provides an opportunity to explore the theme through abstract art and inspirational quotes. If you can, try to create a painting based on a quote before group time to show as an example. Having an example sometimes helps hesitant artists understand the project more clearly.

The quotes provided at the end of this article were found at www.followyourdreams.com/courage.html. Check out the site for additional quotes on courage or other topics.

Materials

18"x24" watercolor paper— one sheet per person
brushes
water
acrylic or watercolor paints
quotations printed and cut out separately
black poster board or matte board for mounting
example of project if possible

background music (new age, or instrumental)

Project

1. Begin the group with paper and paints on tables. Open a discussion about courage: What does the word courage mean to you? Can you give examples of when you have been courageous? Can you give examples of when you have been afraid? How does fear feel to you? How does overcoming a fear feel to you? Can you think of a fear you have faced and overcome?

2. Pass out slips of paper with the provided quotations. After each person picks one, discuss what the quote may mean to him or her.

3. With color and movement, ask each person to think about the meaning of the quote they received, and ask them to create an image that reflects the feeling of the words. For example, I may receive the quote "Do the thing you are afraid to do and the death of fear is certain." — Ralph Waldo Emerson. I may choose to do a painting in which fear will be portrayed as a monster and I have tamed it! Or fear will be painted as black and courage to overcome it will be painted in bright orange rays of the sun. An image of the quote can be made either abstractly or as a representation. Encourage artists to fill the entire white space of the paper with colors. Show your example if available.

4. Allow 15 to 20 minutes to work.

5. When complete and with the consent of the artist, share paintings and the thoughts behind them with the group.

6. Mount pieces on black poster or matte board if possible, and display with the quote.

Facing and overcoming our fears is a difficult thing to do. Courage is within us all. We all must believe we can rise to whatever challenges we face… the help and understanding of our friends will make us even that much stronger.

Quotes

- Do not fear mistakes — there are none. Miles Davis
- One learns by doing a thing; for though you think you know it, you have no certainty until you try. Sophocles
- Do the thing you are afraid to do and the death of fear is certain. Ralph Waldo Emerson
- The best thing about the future is that it only comes one day at a time. Abraham Lincoln
- Every exit is an entry somewhere else. Tom Stoppard
- One sees great things from the valley, only small things from the peak. G. K. Chesterton
- It is not because things are difficult that we do not dare; it is because we do not dare that things are difficult. Seneca
- Trust that still, small voice that says, "This might work and I'll try it." Diane Mariechild
- Life shrinks and expands in proportion to one's courage. Anais Nin
- You must do the thing you think you cannot do. Eleanor Roosevelt
- Once we make our decision, all things will come to us. Auspicious signs are not a superstition, but a confirmation. They are a response. Ming-Dao Deng
- The only way to pass any test is to take the test. Anonymous
- If you are not living on the edge, you take up too much room. Native American saying

Variation of 12

Size	**4 to 12**
Functioning	**high to medium**
Time	**30 to 40 minutes**
Purpose	**group interaction, cooperation, gross motor skills, color and shape identification, art history**

The famous Russian painter, Wassily Kandinsky, inspired the following project. Some credit Kandinsky with the birth of abstract art and he was at the head of the movement in New York in the 1940s and 1950s. His works are best known for their bright, beautiful colors and geometric or abstract design. Bold, bright, and graphic is the look that this final piece will have, when you combine separate paintings into one large mural.

Materials

canvas panels, pre-primed, 8"x10" or 9"x12", a total of twelve canvases
large paint brushes
water containers
acrylic paints
table coverings

Preparation

1. With the assistance of your group members or other volunteers cover the twelve panels in a solid color: three panels in black, three panels in red, three panels in yellow, and three panels in purple or blue.

2. Paint a flat, complete primer application over the panels and allow them to dry completely before group time.

Project

1. Begin a discussion of abstract art. Show examples of Kandinsky's works.
2. Ask each artist to select a colored panel and one color of acrylic paint. Instruct them to paint a geometric shape of their choosing as large as they can on the panel. Fill in the entire shape with the chosen color.
3. When all artists have completed one panel, ask each to do another (if there are fewer than twelve participants) until all panels have a geometric shape in differing colors on them.
4. When dry, allow the artists to choose one panel with a geometric shape on it. It doesn't have to be one that they painted themselves; it could be anyone's. Once selected, ask them to choose a contrasting or complimentary color and to paint the inside of the

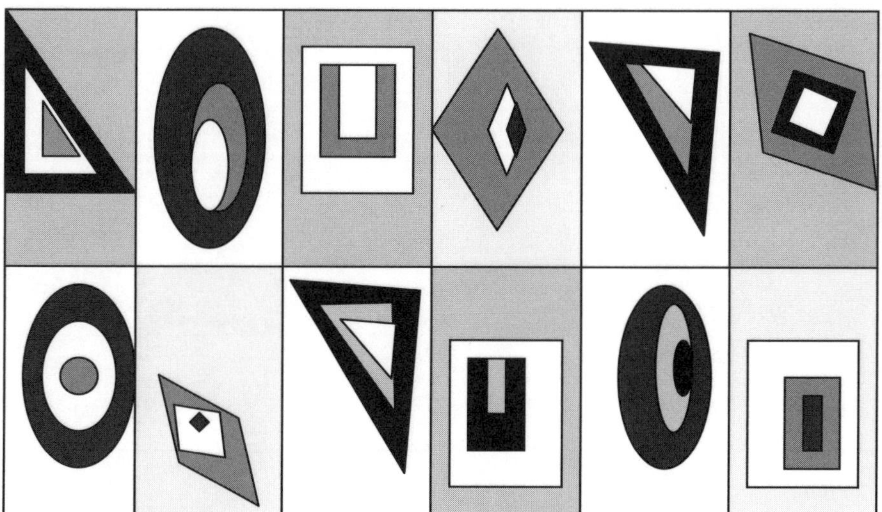

Figure 10. Variation of 12

geometric shape that color, leaving at least an inch of the original paint showing around the edge. (Show by example to give them the idea.)

5. Continue in the same manner until all the shapes are filled in with another bold color.

6. Again, ask artists to select another panel, which now has the two colors and the background color. Choosing another color, ask them to paint that color inside the last shape, again, leaving a portion of the last color showing.

7. Continue until all panels are complete.

8. Once all are complete and dry, clear the worktable and lay out the panels in various ways until the group is satisfied with the arrangement. You should have a bold and abstract mural featuring bright colors and shapes. (See Figure 10.)

9. To display, attach to a smooth wall surface with double sided Velcro tape.

Rothko Inspired Pastels

Size	**6 to 8**
Functioning	**high to medium level (lower level clients may find the pastels difficult to work with)**
Time	**30 minutes**
Purpose	**art education, creativity, fine motor skills**

Mark Rothko was an American painter of the abstract expressionist movement. He, like Kandinsky, was best known for bold, simple, abstract compositions done during the 1950s and 1960s.

Although he worked in paint, his work often has a faded and blurred-out look reminiscent of pastel chalk work. The following project challenges high level clients to work boldly in pastel chalk to create simplified yet beautiful abstract pieces.

NOTE: The use of pastel chalks can be frustrating for artists who are "perfectionists" or don't like to get their hands messy, so give them the option to wear gloves or wrap their chalks with tissue paper to help address this issue. Chalks can be easily blended and faded with the finger, but, again, you may want to offer tissue paper for your clients to blend their colors with instead.

Materials

pastel chalk in a variety of colors
colored charcoal or pastel paper in earth tones (browns, taupe, tan, aqua, green, etc.), 9"x12" sheets or larger depending on the gross motor skills of your group
spray fixative (use in a well-ventilated area away from clients)
rubber gloves or tissue (optional)

examples of Mark Rothko's work

Project

1. Discuss the abstract work of Mark Rothko. Show examples of some of his rectangular pieces like *Orange and Yellow* (1956), *Blue, Untitled* (1960), *Orange, Red* (1961), or *Number 12* (1951).

2. Pass out paper and place in the portrait orientation. Have pastel chalks at artist's places.

Figure 11. Rothko Inspired Pastel

3. Discuss the use of pastel chalks. On a sample piece of paper, demonstrate how a light application of chalk can be laid down and blended out with the finger or a tissue.
4. Ask your artists to select a color of chalk and to roughly draw out a rectangle at the top one-third of their paper. Fill in the rectangle loosely (do not strive for a solid coverage of the paper) and blend the edges out with a tissue to soften.
5. Create another larger rectangle at the bottom of the paper in a different color. Fill and blend as they had the first.
6. As an accent, your clients may opt to add a band of color between the two rectangles if desired. (See Figure 11.) If they choose to do so, cover the bottom rectangle with paper so as not to smear it on their arm or clothing.
7. When complete, step away from clients and spray their work lightly with a chalk fixative to finish off the piece and keep the chalk from smearing.
8. When all pieces are complete, lay them out on the table side by side. Ask each artist to talk about the mood created by his or her piece simply by the choice of colors and the muted application.
9. Title each piece and display separately or as a group.

NOTE: This process can also be done by choosing different geometric shapes, as a collage project, or on canvas with paint!

Hubba, Hubba, Hubble

Size	**6 to 8**
Functioning	**medium to high (lower level clients may find the pastels difficult to work with)**
Time	**30 minutes**
Purpose	**creativity, abstract thinking, mental stimulation, fine motor skills, social interaction**

The Hubble space telescope has offered mankind unbelievable views of breathtaking stellar beauty. Strangely enough, the new photos that arrive from the telescope end up on page eight of the newspaper, or don't get published at all! However, the Internet offers people endless opportunities to keep up to date with the latest images and to download photos for other uses.

The following project utilizes Hubble photographs as inspiration for pastel chalk creations. It also provides the opportunity for clients who may have limited access to the Internet to see the new space discoveries and discuss space exploration in general.

Materials

black drawing paper (9"x12")
pastel chalks
spray fixative (use in a well-ventilated area away from clients)
Hubble space telescope images
rubber gloves or tissue
black matte board for display of images
smocks or aprons if available

viewfinders (Cut a 3"x3" square in the middle of an 8"x11" piece of paper. Slide the viewfinder over images to select areas of interest.)
background music (new age, soothing)

Preparation

Log onto www.Hubblesite.org and go to the "gallery" section of the site. Investigate the showcases of "stars" and "nebula" images. Look for about ten or so abstract looking photos. To download them onto your computer or disc, click on the thumbnail image. Then you can right click on the larger image, go to "save picture as," and choose a folder on your hard drive. Once downloaded, print them out for group use.

Project

1. Begin the group with black paper set in place and pastels available
2. Distribute Hubble photographs. Discuss space exploration and the new images that we see from NASA projects like Hubble. How far do they think mankind can go in space exploration? Would they ever like to travel to another planet?
3. Ask artists to choose one photo that they would like to use for inspiration for a drawing.
4. Once selected, give artists viewfinders and encourage them to move the viewfinder over the photo until they find a pleasing composition from which to work.
5. Briefly instruct them on how to use pastel chalks. Note that the blending of the chalk is desirable and members shouldn't worry about the "messiness" of the chalk. Any blurring that may occur can only enhance the look of the final piece.
6. Help roll up sleeves or provide smocks or aprons if clients are concerned about getting dirty.

7. Allow 20 minutes to work on the pieces. Have soothing music playing in background.

8. Once complete, step away from client area and lightly spray-fix the chalk drawings.

9. Go around the group and look at each person's impression of the Hubble photograph. Title if desired.

10. Display matted pieces along with the inspirational photographs. Include titles and some information on the discussion among group members regarding space discoveries.

Sticky Situations

Size	**6 to 8**
Functioning	**all levels (with some adaptations)**
Time	**30 minutes**
Purpose	**abstract art experience, fun, creativity, fine and gross motor skills**

This project invites the artist to experience an easy art technique with success guaranteed. It is an abstract process including three steps: taping, painting, and removing tape. It can be done in one or two sessions, dependent upon your group's speed of execution and the degree of difficulty they choose.

Materials

10"x14" canvas-like painting panels or any pre-primed hard backed painting canvas (available at most arts/crafts stores)
acrylic paints in a variety of colors, watered down slightly
brushes
water containers
artist tape for canvases (Scotch makes some, but you can also use painter's tape available at hardware stores) Have several rolls available for artists to share.

Project

1. Distribute painting panels and tape.
2. Talk about abstract art and how fine art doesn't always have to be representational. It can be spontaneous and fun and still be aesthetically pleasing!

3. Invite the artists to stretch and apply long pieces of the tape across their panels. Let them know that whatever is taped will be white in the final piece. Encourage them to crisscross, overlap, and stretch tape from one edge of the canvas to another.
4. Once all the panels are taped up (about seven to nine pieces should do it), leaving plenty of space for color, have artists select a few paints to apply and blend together on the canvas. Clients may swirl the colors together or paint large sections solidly.
5. Allow the canvases to dry somewhat before removing the tape. (This is a good time to clean up brushes!)
6. Assist artists with removing the tape from the canvas to reveal an abstract display of colors and lines.
7. Ask each artist to show their piece to other group members and to give it a title.
8. Display.

Adaptations

1. You may want to pre-tape a larger canvas to use as a group project with lower level clients, focusing on gross motor skills, fun, and discussion.
2. You can invite your group to re-tape the piece once thoroughly dry and paint over the entire remainder of the canvas with a solid black color to give you a stained glass type appearance.

Pollack Inspired Drip Art

Size	**6 to 8**
Functioning	**high to medium**
Time	**two sessions; 20 to 30 minutes each**
Purpose	**art education, spontaneity, self-expression, gross motor skills, discussion**

Jackson Pollack was a leader in the abstract impressionist movement of the 1940s and 1950s. Giant canvases filled with dripped and splashed paints were his trademark and made him one of the most widely recognizable artists of that era. *Lucifer, Mural,* and *Untitled 1946* are some of his better known pieces that offer the viewer rich colors, grand gestured design, and intriguing composition.

In the following two-session project, high to medium cognitive functioning clients are asked to learn about Pollack's work through experiencing his technique. We use pre-stretched and primed canvases and acrylic paints to replicate Pollack's style, although a larger group piece or smaller individual pieces may also be explored. No paintbrushes are used here, as we do not want clients to apply the paint directly. I recommend short dowels, or paint stirring sticks, but old rulers or whatever you can find to use to splash or drip paint is fine. As paint will be dispensed into plastic cups (to encourage a heavier application), monitor your clients while working, so that no one forgets the cups are filled with paint and not coffee! (Please use clear plastic cups, if possible, to help clients see clearly what they have before them.)

If range of motion is a consideration for your group, cover the floor with a drip cloth, and place canvases on the floor to the side of the artist. Place paints and sticks on bedside tables and be prepared to rotate the canvas as requested.

Do a little research on Jackson Pollack, and provide color samples of his work for your group. Look online (www.allposters.com has some good examples) or at your local library for more information.

Materials

acrylic paints in a variety of colors
12" dowels or paint sticks
14"x18" canvas panels (pre-primed and stretched), one per person
table covering and painting smocks for clients
12-oz. clear plastic cups for paints
examples of Jackson Pollack works
background music

Preparation

1. Have tables covered and canvases at each artist place.
2. Dispense acrylic paints into cups. Prepare a set of like colors such as red, brown, black, and orange, or blue, greens, purples, and magentas, etc., to give to artists. I recommend limiting and pre-selecting the colors here to give your artists a good start and to allow them to concentrate on the movement of the paint, rather than on the color selection. Also, by grouping colors together into aesthetically pleasing complements, you are insuring a more cohesive and beautiful final piece for each artist.

Project

Session one

1. Begin the group with a discussion of Jackson Pollack's work as described above. Show samples of his work to the group and discuss. Invite members of the group to discover more about Pollack by immersing themselves in his art technique.
2. Ask artists to select a color set of three to four colors, all including black. Artists may also choose just black and white.

3. Once colors have been selected and dispensed, give artists the paint sticks and encourage them to apply the color to the canvas in a loose and spontaneous manner by dripping the paint on with sticks or by pouring it sweepingly over the canvas. Again, reference examples of Pollack's work and encourage a gradual buildup of paint on the canvas. Remind artists to be mindful of other people's work and to limit their "flinging" of paint to their own workspace.
4. Work for 20 minutes and allow the pieces to dry until the next session.

Session two

1. Revisit the theme of Jackson Pollack's work. Explain that clients may now look again at their pieces from the last session and add to it using the same color palette or an additional color. Remind the artist that they want to fill every space of their canvas with the color, line, and movement of the applied paint.
2. Allow another 15 to 20 minutes of work time as needed.
3. When artists are done, ask them to title their piece and share it with the rest of the group.
4. Display all pieces together with an explanation of the inspiration for the group.

This two-session process will allow members to experience not only the spontaneity of abstract art, but to also realize the consideration given to composition, application, and design of the work. This process should be fun and result in visually exciting works of art. You might also try this process on canvases painted a solid black. Working on a black background requires less effort to "fill" the space with color and can cut your group time in half for clients with short attention spans.

Miscellaneous

The following projects utilize different art media to explore various cultures, traditional arts, and using myths and lore as inspiration for creativity. They may use specialty items, such as decorative papers, papier-mâché forms, or other things that may require a little more planning on your part. Plan ahead and don't be afraid to splurge on a few art items occasionally. It's exciting for artists to use different types of canvas or backgrounds for their art making process and can re-energize a group that may be stuck in the "painting of the week" mode. Don't be afraid to really delve into a theme with your group. If the art piece is centered on the orient, feel free to expand on that idea by providing ethnic foods, music, and clothing to help create the mood. Your art group is an opportunity to grow and explore, not just in art media, but in all aspects of life. You provide the stimulation, and you never know whose imagination you may excite!

Celebrating the Orient

Size	**6 to 8**
Functioning	**high to medium; low with adaptations**
Time	**30 minutes**
Purpose	**cultural exploration, fine motor skills, discussion**

The Eastern culture has a tradition of writing happy wishes on red paper as part of a New Year celebration. We don't need to wait until the calendar changes to think about making changes in our lives and our mental attitudes, and this project highlights that fact.

We take the idea of the New Year's resolution and the Chinese custom of "happy wishes" and use it to give our clients an opportunity to think about making changes and committing to those changes at any time of the year.

I use a specialty paper for this project that is decorated with Chinese calligraphy and offers a nice element of the Far East in a simple manner. You can find paper such as this through your fine arts supply store or at a craft store location. I suggest using these specific supplies to create the rich beauty of traditional Chinese art and textures.

This project is most successful with high to medium level clients, but may be done with lower cognitive level clients as well. You need to precut and glue the envelopes, and focus on the discussion of happy wishes, and the process of decorating the front side of the envelope.

Materials

orient inspired decorative paper
envelope template (Figure 12)
small twigs the size of toothpicks
heavy red threads or string

hot glue
solid glue sticks
scissors
small sheets of red paper
black writing markers

Project

1. Begin the group with a discussion of resolutions. Are resolutions only for New Year's Eve or can we make resolutions or set goals at all times of the year? Talk about how today's project is inspired by the Eastern tradition of holding in high regard our resolutions, happy wishes, and goals by treating these thoughts with honor and esteem. Discuss the use of red here as part of the custom to insure a bright and happy future (red is seen as a bright and happy color).

2. Place the sheets of decorative paper in the middle of the table. Talk about the beautiful forms of Chinese calligraphy. Allow each person to select one piece.

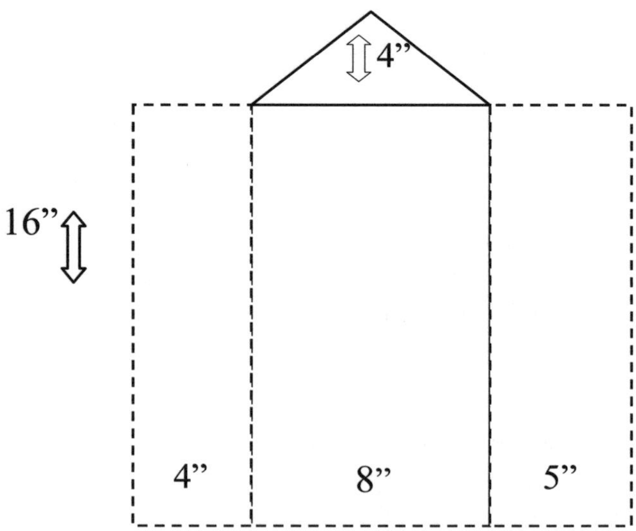

Figure 12. Template for Envelope

3. Trace the envelope template onto it and cut out as shown in Figure 12. (Or do this ahead of group time if your clients will be unable, or if time will not allow for this step.)
4. Once cut, fold as shown in Figure 13 and apply glue from solid glue stick to the one inch of overlap paper (right side) and the bottom edge of paper, and seal envelope.
5. Next, bring out the metallic papers and tear or cut it into strips to decorate the front (non-seam) side of the envelope in a collage type fashion. Layering the papers in a linear fashion can bring exciting highlights of color without cluttering the look of the envelope.
6. Hot glue twigs to one area of the front as an accent. Twigs may be "bundled" together with red thread or string before gluing.
7. When done, fold the top flap over. Hot glue a twig horizontally on the flap. Hot glue string, under a scrap of paper, onto the envelope below it to act as a closure. String will be wrapped

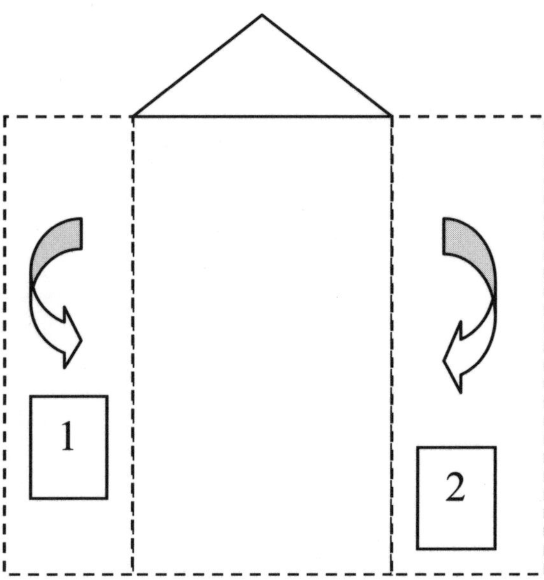

Figure 13. Folding the Envelope

around the twig on the flap to close as in Figure 14.

8. Finally, ask each person to write a resolution or goal on the small piece of red paper. This resolution or goal should be something achievable and meaningful to them. Artists may choose to share their resolutions with the group at this time.

9. Place the resolution/goal into the envelope and seal it with the string closure.

By creating a beautiful envelope to hold the resolution we are giving that goal or thought special significance. The envelope, itself a work of art, may be left in plain view in the client's room, as a daily reminder to work towards meeting the goal or resolve.

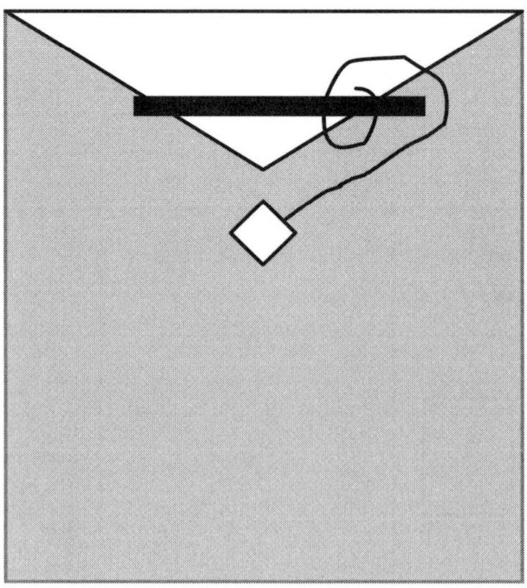

Figure 14. Finished Envelope

Fruits of Creativity

Size	**6 to 8**
Functioning	**high to medium**
Time	**30 to 40 minutes (could be done in two shorter sessions)**
Purpose	**discussion, creativity, fine motor skills**

The act of the Harvest is a theme that crosses most cultures and generations. Mankind knows the importance of gathering the bounty from the earth for continuation of life; therefore, this important endeavor has been recreated in all art forms since the beginning of time.

The following project was inspired by the story of Pomona, the Roman goddess of fruit and fertility and patron of gardens and fruit orchards.

The story reads that Pomona was a beautiful and loving goddess, sought after by many gods. After much convincing, Vertumnus, the god of seasons and the growth of plants, won her heart. Their union seemed to be ideal, since it coupled the cycle of seasons and the fruition of trees and crops.

This story is to be used as an inspiration for the following project, which marries known art techniques (painting) with an unusual "canvas."

You will be using papier-mâché apple forms, which are available at most craft stores. (You can also order them online at www.dcccrafts.com. DCC Crafts also offers an apple-shaped papier-mâché box which could also be used if fine motor skills are a problem with your clients.)

Having a volunteer or assistant to help you and the artists during this process is very beneficial, as artists may need help using materials or manipulating the apple form.

Materials

papier-mâché apples, one per person, medium to large size
acrylic paints
small brushes
water
metallic paints
table coverings
glitter and glue, small magazine pictures, Mod Podge, ribbons, small artificial flowers and hot glue
background music
fresh apples cut up for the aroma and to snack on later (make sure to check for any conflicts with dietary or swallowing guidelines for your clients.)

Project

1. Begin the group with a discussion of the harvest season. Talk about the Roman myth of Pomona and Vertumnus.

2. Pass out papier-mâché apples. In honor of the story of Pomona (apple mother), invite the artists to create beautiful paintings on the apple form. They are not to just paint the apple red or green, but to think of the apple as a canvas for which they can create any type of painting, abstract or representational. (Have a sample to show if you can!)

3. Dispense paints and brushes and make sure clients look at all the colors available to them before beginning. Once the creativity begins to flow, your clients may ask for additional supplies, such as glitter and glue, small magazine pictures, and Mod Podge (good for lower level clients), ribbons, small artificial flowers, and hot glue (please assist), or anything else they can think of.

4. Assist in the creative process as necessary. If some of your clients are unable to hold the apple as they work, use sandbags to rest the apple in for stability or use the apple shaped papier-mâché boxes instead. Encourage artists to work an area and let it

dry so they do not smear it as they go. This process could take two group periods, if you choose.

5. When all apples are finished, discuss the varieties of work that have been done. Display apples hanging from a branch or suspended from display case or area.

6. Share apple snack to end the group.

Money, Money, Money

Size	**8 to 10**
Functioning	**high to medium; low with adaptations**
Time	**30 minutes**
Purpose	**discussion, reality orientation, creativity, fine motor skills**

Money is pocket art that we use as a means of trade. If you have ever had a few dollars in your pockets long enough to look closely at it, you discovered that currency contains beautifully detailed images that tell a story about the culture that created it. If you have traveled outside the United States, you saw that many countries have currency made up of beautiful images and many colors!

The following project allows clients of many cognitive and physical functioning levels to address money for its artistic, rather than monetary, value.

Materials

- black and white photocopies of different currency (Go to www.Banknotes.com for really great worldwide currency art!); include a variety of U.S. bills, plus some foreign currency
- colored pencils
- glue sticks
- black paper 12"x14"
- black matte boards
- scissors

Project

1. Begin a discussion about money. What is the first thing they think of when you say the word "money?" (Paying bills, past wages, prices going up?)

2. Talk about the art of money. Have they ever really looked closely at U.S. bills? Have they studied the intricate details of the images and portraits? Have they ever seen foreign money? Show pictures of foreign bills from books or a personal collection. What can you learn about a culture by its money?

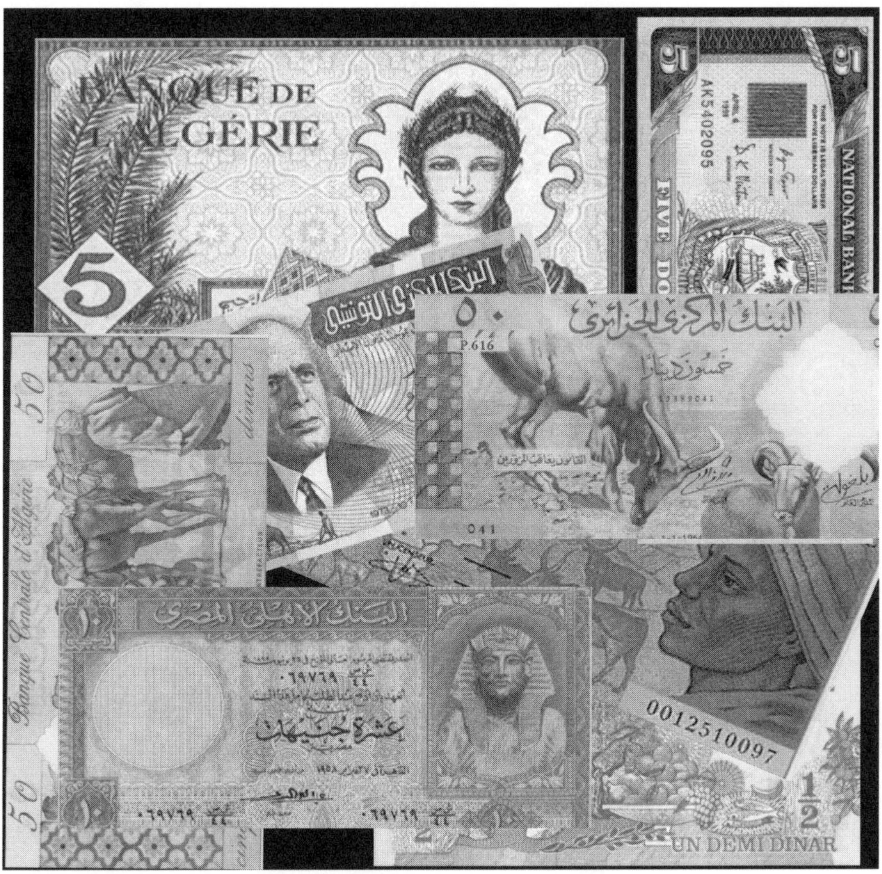

Figure 15. Money, Money, Money

3. Place the black and white photocopied money you have prepared out on the tables. Photocopy many different types on a page and do not pre-cut. (It is easier to color to the edge of the bill if you have some surrounding paper to draw out towards.)
4. Using the colored pencils, lightly color over the money. You can use several colors on each bill. Fill in only certain detail areas or color the whole bill in one color. Each person should complete two to three 8.5"x11" photocopied sheets of bills.
5. When complete, assist in cutting the bills apart.
6. Using the colored money as collage materials, ask the artists to arrange the bills onto the black paper, gluing down as they go. Encourage them to overlap the bills and put them on in a disorderly fashion.
7. When complete, matte with a black matte board. You should end up with a hand colored, black and white photograph-looking collage! (Figure 15)

Options

1. You may also print out colored versions of the money from www.Banknotes.com, pre-cut them, and use this as collage material for all level groups.
2. Feed 8.5"x11" pieces of student grade watercolor paper through your computer printer to give the copies more of a real money feel! (Set printing options for a heavier paper setting.)
3. If you know of someone with a banknote collection, show the artists first hand what the money looks and feels like!

NOTE: Photocopied and computer generated currency images are not to be used for trade!

Overall, this process should help open participants eyes to the art that surrounds us and is many times overlooked.

Closer Looks

Size	**6 to 8**
Functioning	**high to medium**
Time	**30 to 40 minutes (may be done in two sessions)**
Purpose	**creativity, using new art media, self-expression, self-awareness**

This project uses a digital or instant camera and copy machine for a dramatic self-portrait image. It asks clients to think about their most favorite physical attribute and to use that feature as the basis for a meaningful art piece.

Materials

camera
copy machine
colored pencils (optional)
black writing marker
dry glue sticks
black poster board
scissors
background music

Project

1. Talk about physical features. Ask your artists to identify one feature that they think is their best or favorite. (Eyes, hands, feet, ears, hair, or bald spots!)
2. Using the camera, take a close-up photo of that feature.

3. Print out the photo and have the artist crop the photo so that the selected feature is all that remains.
4. On the photo copy machine, copy the image (you may want to enlarge it somewhat) so that the artist has six to ten images to work with.
5. Images may be hand colored using a light application of colored pencil if they choose.
6. On a piece of black poster board (cut to the artist's chosen size), instruct the artists to arrange the images onto the board in a linear pattern.
7. Looking at their pieces, can they think of a title, or words that they would like to add to it? If so, they may write that across the collage with the black marker, or save it and display the piece with the title on a card.

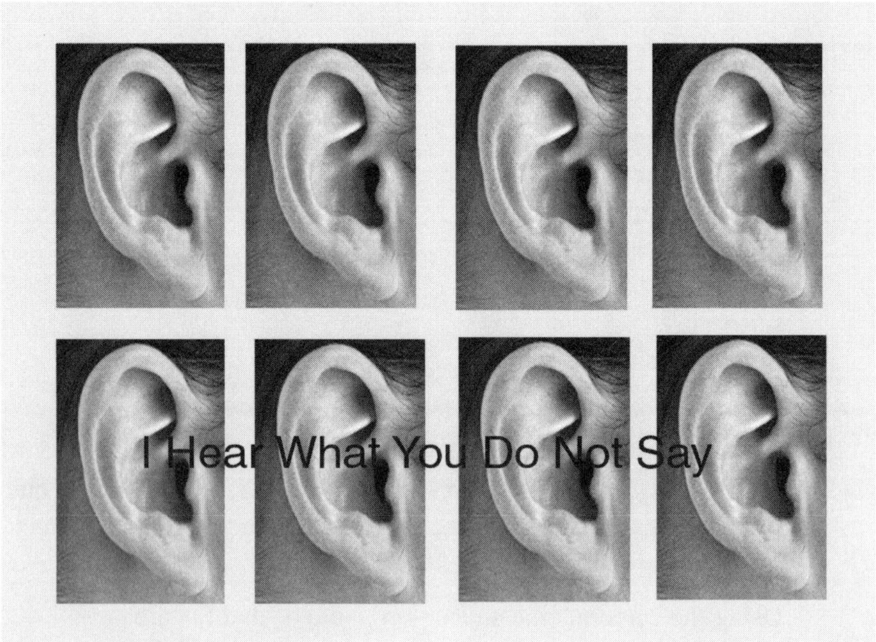

Figure 16. Closer Look 1

Save time to look at each person's finished collage. As a group, discuss the feeling of the piece and what kind of emotional reactions it may elicit.

The finished image can be humorous or powerfully telling, but it is guaranteed to turn heads and make people stop to look. (Figure 16 and Figure 17)

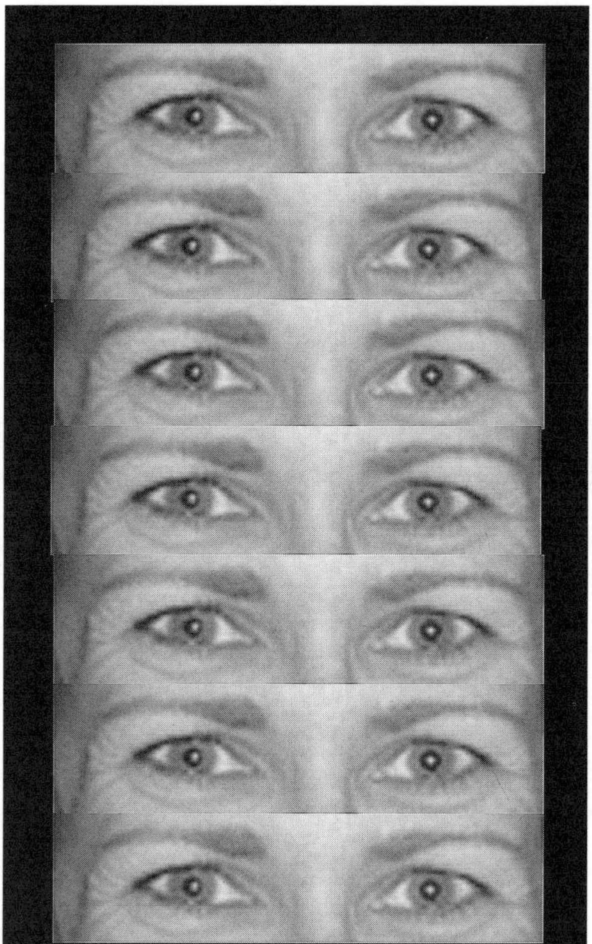

Figure 17. Closer Look 2

Wedgies

Size	**4 to 6**
Functioning	**all levels**
Time	**20 to 30 minutes**
Purpose	**fun, creative expression, group interaction, discussion**

This project utilizes segments of a circle and a limited paint selection to provide the opportunity for self-expression, group dynamics, and fun for all levels of clients. It provides the opportunity to discuss feelings of belonging and acknowledgment of our differences. I use oil pastels in the original plan as they cover well, are more age appropriate than wax crayons, and, with their creamy texture, have the ability to blend. Please see the end of the project for other options.

Materials

22"x28" white poster board
oil pastels (need several boxes and as wide an assortment of colors as possible)
22"x28" black poster board
spray mount adhesive or dry glue
light music playing in background

Preparation

1. Cut your 22"x28" white poster board into a large circle.
2. Next, divide the circle into wedges based upon the number of members in your group. For example, if your group has six members, the circle should be divided into six pie-like segments.

3. Divide oil pastels into different color schemes. For example, one artist will get all the shades of red (pink, flesh, and red); one will get all the shades of blue, green, etc. Include white and black with all so artists may create their own shades by blending.

Project

1. Distribute white poster board wedges and oil pastels before group members arrive.
2. When members arrive, let them know that the challenge today is to fill their segment with as many shades of the same color as they can. They should use line and shape for interest. The music should dictate the mood and they should just create freely and joyfully. They must fill in all the white areas of their segment. Have an example to help them understand that the piece will be most likely an abstract, color exploration.
3. Allow 20 minutes or so to work.
4. When all are complete, lay the black poster board in the center of the worktables, and invite members to lay their segments onto the board to create the circle.
5. When the circle is complete, talk about the different styles and colors everyone used. Does each segment indicate a mood or theme? As a whole circle, do they create a different mood? How does the circle, with all its different parts, relate to the group members and all their differences?
6. Dry glue or spray glue the circle onto the black background. As a group, can they think of a title for the piece?

Adaptations

1. For lower level groups, use watercolor paper and paints. Lay flat to dry before assembling into a circle.

2. For higher level groups this could be done on a gessoed (meaning prepared for painting) Masonite board (cut into a circle and segmented with a saw) and painted on with acrylic paints. Each segment should be painted to reflect something about the artist's personality using all colors available.

NOTE: Pre-gessoed Masonite boards are available at arts and crafts stores or through Saxarts.com. Ask your facilities maintenance man to cut it for you.

Surreal Experiences

Size	**6 to 10**
Functioning	**high and medium**
Time	**session one: 25 to 30 minutes** **session two: 30 minutes**
Purpose	**art education, fun, creativity, exploration of new mixed media process, self-expression**

Surrealistic art is an unusual art process that came about in 1920 in Paris. It literally means "super realism" and might be best known for the dreamlike images painted by Salvador Dali during the mid 20th century. One of its basic characteristics would be the unusual arrangement of dissimilar items or themes.

We achieve a surreal-like image in this project by combining artist-created linear or landscape designs and magazine photographs. It is meant to be a fun, challenging way to introduce artists to this kind of expressive art.

Materials

watercolor paper 18"x24" (can be halved if you choose)
watercolor paints or high intensity inks
water containers
paper towels
brushes
magazine photographs
dry glue sticks
samples of Salvador Dali's work (look for *Meditative Rose* (1958) or *The Elephants* (1948) as good examples)

Preparation

Find large colorful magazine images of unusual items, such as tools, make up, bathroom fixtures, cars, large blossoms, etc. Cut out these images, isolating the image from the background. For example, if you are cutting out an image of a toilet from a bathroom advertisement, cut out only the toilet and not the tiled floor, the sink, or anything else. (NOTE: the more fun and unusual images you can find, the more fun and unusual the final pieces will be.)

Project

Session one

1. Have watercolor paints or inks, brushes, and water containers at each artist's place.
2. Begin a discussion of Salvador Dali's work. Show examples. Ask members to dissect the pieces somewhat. What do they include? (Landscape, plus some unusual item that seems out of place.) Do the paintings seem dreamlike to them?
3. Tell your artists that they will be constructing a surrealistic art piece over the next two sessions.
4. With the watercolor paints and paper, encourage participants to create a beautiful, colorful, and linear landscape filling their entire paper surface. They should make it as colorful and unusual as they want, but should keep it basically simple.
5. Allow 15 to 20 minutes to work.
6. Allow paintings to dry and flatten under heavy objects until the following group session.

Session two

1. Place the dried and flattened landscape paintings at each client's place and lay all the magazine photographs within reach of group members.

2. Remind group members about the discussion of surrealistic art. Show examples again if need be.
3. Invite them to look through the magazine images you have provided and to pick one that appeals the most to them because of its humor, colors, shape, or personal interest.
4. Once selected, have the artist place their image on their landscape painting. Once the area has been selected, glue in place. (Figure 18)
5. When all pieces are done, begin a discussion about Dali's work. Invite members to show their final pieces, select titles, and discuss their feelings about the project and the finished product.
6. Display with an explanation of the process.

Overall this process is meant to be fun and educational. It is usually met with lots of giggles and creative ideas.

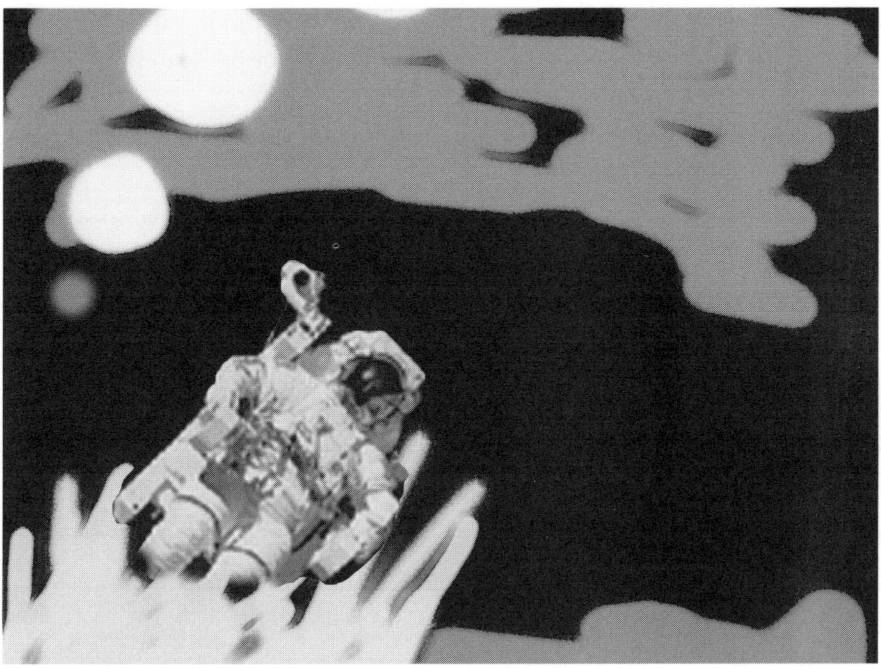

Figure 18. Surreal Experiences

Signs and Symbols

Size	**6 to 8**
Functioning	**high to medium**
Time	**20 minutes**
Purpose	**discussion, self-expression, creativity, gross motor skills**

Signs and symbols confront us every day. We take for granted our ability to substitute an icon, shape, or color for a word, and the degree in which signs and symbols simplify our communications. There are so many symbolic meanings for everyday thoughts, feelings, and items that there are several books and web sites devoted to the definition of them. For this process I researched symbols on www.symbols.com. You can find lots of different web sites on the same subject by searching online under the term "symbols."

The following project uses a discussion of signs and symbols as a starting point for a graphic art piece.

Materials

white poster board, one per person
oil pastels or acrylic paints and brushes
chalkboard or large sheet of paper for brainstorming symbols
collection of lesser known symbols (see end of project or go to www.symbols.com)
black marker

Project

1. Distribute white poster board and oil pastels

2. Begin a discussion of everyday signs and symbols. On the chalkboard or paper, draw out the symbols discussed. They may include the dollar sign, treble clef (music symbol), stop or yield sign shapes, barber shop pole, wedding ring, black arm band, yellow ribbons, etc.
3. Discuss some lesser-known symbols (as seen below).
4. Ask each group member to select a symbol they would like to embellish for their art piece.
5. Using the oil pastels (or acrylic paint option) instruct the artists to either create one giant representation of the symbol they have

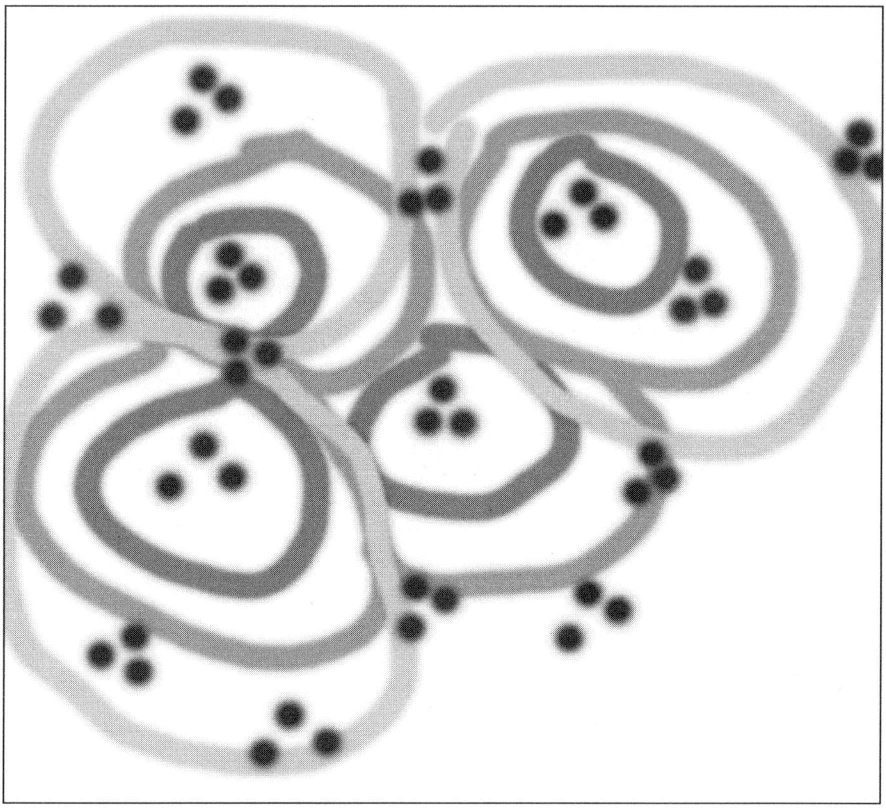

Figure 19. Signs and Symbols

chosen, or they may fill their paper with a repeated image over and over to create a random design. (Figure 19)

6. Encourage the blending of color and the thickening of the symbol beyond the linear representation. For example, if the artist has chosen the dollar sign, they should embellish the basic shape through the use of additional colors, decorations, and stylizing to make it their own.

7. When all are complete, discuss the decisions behind their sign or symbol selection and share resulting artwork.

Other symbology

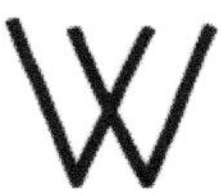

"Viva" Live!

Maltese cross or Cross of Promise. Stands for loyalty, piety, generosity, courage, honor, and glory.

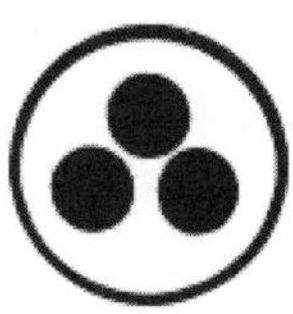

Hobo sign of protection, faith, love, and hope

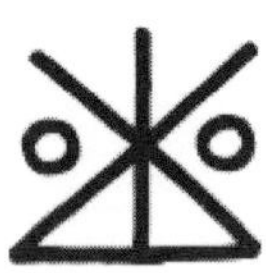

Sign for Family

Guided Stories

There is value in story telling and meditation. Taking a client to a safe, imaginative place with words so that they can further create and explore is a useful tool in therapy. It helps to break "artists block," or can be used to challenge a client who has repeatedly taken safe routes by creating in one media or in one style. You can summon someone to look out at the world through a perspective other than his or her own, to increase empathy for others, or to explore a conflictive relationship among peers. It should be used with high to medium cognitive level clients who will be able to respond, not in frustration or confusion, but with imagination and fervor.

Please don't confuse the following stories with guided imagery, which could also be defined as directed meditation or daydreaming. In its truest sense, guided imagery is used by a trained practitioner to promote relaxation and healing. The stories that we are using here will also do that, as a natural by-product of the art making process. However, no therapeutic intervention should be administered unless you are a trained professional in that modality. During an imagery exercise, a therapist would guide a person in visualizations with a specific healing purpose in mind. The purpose of our guided stories is to challenge and inspire.

We use brief "stories" for clients to reflect upon and to respond to in any artistic way. They can create a drawing, painting, or poem in response to the suggested reflection. This is a great way to challenge the imagination muscle and can be used within a group, in an "art studio" setting to help break artist block or to give a client a place to start for unique and creative expression. I have listed some guided stories here. Use these as starting points for more expanded art process, to further build a group around, or as intended here, as a springboard for creation for your clients. After each story is a recommended media approach and information on processing the resulting piece.

A tortoise shell reflects the beauty of nature, as well as an image of the life of the soul beneath it. If you had a shell, what would it look like?

Recommended media: Oil pastels or markers on drawing paper. You might want to have photographs or pictures of tortoise shells to demonstrate the repeated design and pattern found in nature.

Processing notes: If the client could not draw a shell or drew one with holes or made out of flimsy materials, it may indicate feeling vulnerable and insecure. The client could be asked to continue to improve upon the image until it is sturdy and tough — a shell of strength and self-confidence.

If the client drew a vibrant and extravagant shell, he or shee might be known as an individualistic person, one who loves drama and enjoys attention.

The act of drawing a shell of this sort can be very meditative; the client should feel free to lose themselves in the intricacies.

You are standing in a doorway off a busy street on a gray and rainy day. You look down at the rain as it puddles and runs along the street. Listen to the noise around you. What does the raindrop feel as it comes to earth? Does it crash into the concrete or does it rest in the arms of its companions already on the ground? Draw the rain.

Recommended media: Watercolor paints and paper.

Processing notes: This story may show how the client interprets the rain itself. Do they see it as the enemy? Crashing into the ground below in a violent way? This may indicate a feeling of vulnerability and a penchant for feeling the victim.

If they perceived the rain in all its beauty, as a poetic and lovely vision, they may be a person who lives in the moment. They may be said to enjoy the good in everything and be optimistic and poetic in nature.

Imagine yourself driving down a country road on a sunny day — windows open, the air blowing your hair around your face. Looking to your left you see golden rows of corn and a jade blue sky. Grasshoppers jump from unknown places. How do you feel? Draw that feeling.

Recommended media: Oil pastels or acrylic paints for control.

Processing notes: Most responses to this story will be airy, filled with images of freedom, flying, joy, and peace. If, however, you find the story makes the client feel uneasy and lonely, there may be fears of being alone or the client may be uncomfortable with his or her own company and abilities to be out in the world. Encourage clients to be their own best friend, trust themselves, and acknowledge their own worthiness.

You are confronted by a hall of doors. Each door is more magnificent than the last. One door has your name on it. What does the doorway look like?

Recommended media: oil pastels or acrylic paints.

Processing notes: You are asking your clients to create a door that represents themselves. If the door is solid, foreboding, and threatening, they may be saying that they are afraid to let others in. If the door is made with a window, or slats that allow people to see what lies behind, perhaps they are a very open person, who enjoys the company of others and may like meeting new people and experiencing new things. If the door is ornate and showy, they may think highly of themselves. They may value themselves and enjoy others, seeing the very best they have to offer.

You are flying. What colors and shapes do you see beneath you?

Recommended media: Watercolor paints and paper.

Processing notes: This story is meant to allow the clients to create abstractly, with flowing movements for a relaxing experience. If the drawing is a detailed image of objects the client is flying over, the client may be very literal, very detail oriented, or feel unsafe in an unstructured environment.

You are a stone on a beach. You are picked up and bounced across the water. What do you see and feel?

Recommended media: Watercolor paints and paper.

Processing notes: This is an exercise for the imagination. Your clients should be encouraged to explore the colors, the feelings of this story and create without censor. Do they feel being bounced across the water is hurting them? Perhaps that is evidence of fear of the lack of control they might be experiencing in everyday life.

You are in an underwater ship. You stand in the middle of a circular room of portholes. All around you is the life and color of the ocean. You begin to spin, making all the images you see blend together. What does it look like to you?

Recommended media: Watercolor paints and paper or pastel chalks and drawing paper.

Processing note: The clients are encouraged to allow themselves to spontaneously create using the underwater colors of their choosing. They should find freedom in the blending and movement of the process.

You find yourself standing in an open field under a full moon. Everything around you is colored with the midnight darkness. Suddenly a shower of lights falls around you, as if you are in the middle of a field of falling stars. You are unhurt, but mesmerized. What do you see and how do you feel?

Recommended Media: Watercolor paints and paper or pastel chalk and drawing paper.

Processing notes: The image they create from the story of the meteor shower will most likely represent calm, amazement, and a feeling of themselves as part of the universe.

You sway through the air. Looking upon yourself you see not hands and feet, but feathers. You are floating — a feather. You pass through light that shines through a dusty window. You float and dance on small currents of air. What do you see through your eyes?

Recommended media: Watercolor paints and paper.

Processing notes: The response will most likely be a peaceful, airy image. This story can be used as a meditation and to provide an opportunity to relax and feel free.

You are an anchor. To what are you tied? What do you look like?

Recommended media: Oil pastels or markers and paper.

Processing notes: This process lets the clients create a literal interpretation or a more philosophical image. Do they feel heavy, weighted down? Do they fear they may be holding themselves or someone else back? The answer to the question, "to what are you tied?" may be an eye opener. If the client answers a person or a specific situation, and sees that as a negative thing, now may be the time to challenge that bond and to encourage them to develop reasonable goals to address it.

You have the ability to do anything. You are strong and confident and nothing can stop you from achieving what you dream of. What kind of adventure will you take on?

Recommended media: Markers, oil pastels, or watercolor paints and paper.

Processing notes: This is mostly an exercise in imagination. Clients should come away from it feeling refreshed and invigorated.

Chapter 7

Fund Raising

Implementing art groups whose result is a sellable, revenue building product is not the number one priority of a therapeutic art group. However, it is nice to provide an opportunity for your clients to create beautiful gift items for family and friends or to use as part of a craft sale or fund-raiser. Ideally, if you need to create products for a craft sale, prepare enough materials so the artist may take home a finished piece as they create one or two for sale.

The following projects were all groups that I ran without thinking about the end product as a sellable item. However, occasionally a display of client work results in a phone call or two about purchasing items. Facility staff or friends may want to purchase work done by your clients because of the aesthetic beauty of the work or for sentimental reasons, such as love for the artist. Either way, selling client work in a limited way can be rewarding for both the client and the art supply fund.

Art Projects that Make Money

Before you think about selling client–made items you need to have express permission from the client. If I were preparing for a craft sale, I would invite clients to come in to work on items expressly for that purpose. Your artists may be thrilled that you value the quality of their work enough to offer it for sale to others. Make sure that the clients get something in return. A piece to take home for themselves or a thank you card shows them that their time and talents are worth something to you. Confidentiality also needs to be discussed. Do they want their name on the pieces? That choice is up to them. I might also suggest compiling a list of items created by each individual for sale, with a blanket permission signature to sell these items. Any money collected would go back into the art supplies you use for future groups, and your clients can feel good about their contributions.

Below (Figure 20) is a basic permission form you can have your clients sign if they will be contributing artwork for an art sale. Please only include clients who are able to understand that they are donating their time and talent to the fundraising cause. Approaching somewhat confused or forgetful clients with this opportunity may have them scratching their heads and lead to a whole avalanche of miscommunication and confusion regarding the work that they create. I generally invite only high to medium level cognitive functioning clients to this kind of "special workshop" just to avoid complications.

Permission Form

I, (client's name), give my permission for the following items to be sold for fundraising purposes. I donate my time and talent, knowing that any money generated by the sale of the below listed items will be used in the purchase of future art supplies for groups held at this facility.

Signature: ______________________________ date: _________

Figure 20. Permission Form

Silk Scarves

Creating beautiful silk scarves is easier than you think. Today you can find pre-hemmed and prepared scarf blanks and all you need to do is apply the paint or inks! Here are the basic instructions.

Materials

finished silks for painting — 9"x54" silk scarves available through Sax Arts and Crafts (1-800-558-6696)
fabric paint - Jacquard makes some that can be applied with a brush, or use Tie Dye Cords for an easier application
water source
brushes
paper toweling and table covers

Project

1. Cover work surface with paper toweling
2. Lay out scarf blanks.
3. Wet scarves, and apply fabric paint in a loose abstract way. Add water to the paints to create a watercolor painted effect. To use Tie-Dye Cords, lay cords out on silk. Roll silk into a tube with the cords inside. Saturate with water. Press lightly to release dye from cords. Unroll to see a beautiful repeated pattern.
4. Allow scarves to dry and heat set either in a dryer or with an iron applied to the reverse side.

NOTE: Color selection is key to making these scarves sellable. Choose beautiful blues, greens, reds, and violets for the most versatile scarves.

Puzzle Piece Pins

This is a fun and easy way to make glamorous looking art/jewelry on a budget. It uses puzzle pieces as the main surface of the pin. These may be salvaged from the never-ending supply of incomplete puzzles donated to your facility!

Materials

puzzle pieces in good condition
metallic spray paints or acrylic paints in gold, silver, and copper
black spray paint or acrylic paint
paint brushes
hot glue gun
pin backings
black card stock cut into 5"x5" squares
small, natural bird feathers or colored feathers available from your local craft store

Preparation

Spray paint a variety of puzzle pieces (glossy side up) in metallic and black colors, OR hand paint with metallic and black acrylic paints. Let dry.

Project

1. Taking two or three small puzzle pieces of one or two colors, layer them on top of each other slightly and hot glue in place. (Help artists with this part so that they don't burn their fingers.)
2. Hot glue a few feathers to the back so that they stick out from behind the puzzle pieces
3. Hot glue a pin backing onto the back

4. When done, stick the pin through a black piece of card stock to sell and display

Paper Weights

This is a basic collage/nature project that has a Japanese feel to it. It utilizes natural elements to create a beautiful and simple art piece with a function.

Materials

medium sized smooth rocks (about the size of your fist or smaller) found at a beach or garden center.
natural handmade fiber paper in reds, blues, and violets (can be found at a fine arts store or stationary store)
Mod Podge glossy glue/glaze
raffia strings (a colorful, fibrous craft string)
paint brush

Project

1. Wash and dry rocks
2. Focusing on the top, middle portion of the rock, tear small to medium strips of the natural fiber paper, place and overlap papers onto the rock with the Mod Podge glue.
3. When a nice arrangement has been made, coat the entire surface of the rock with the glaze to firmly attach the papers and shine the rock.
4. When dry, take a few pieces of colorful raffia string and wrap around the rock. Tie with a small knot at the top.
5. Sell as art or paper weights!

Abstract Art Uses

Basic Cards

Decorating a basic card blank is easy and fun for all level clients. By simply cutting down abstract art pieces to the correct card-front size, you have beautiful, handmade, unique all-occasion cards to sell. You can glue art pieces onto blank cards kits, available widely at office supply stores (generally to be used with computer generated art or photographs) or at craft stores.

Picture Frames and Mugs Inserts

Again, utilizing scraps from past art projects, you can overlay cardboard picture frame blanks or use them as inserts into plastic craft mugs.

There is such a wide selection of craft projects for you to personalize on the market right now that your imagination and budget are your only limitations.

Chapter 8

Putting it All Together...

My hope for you is that this book will be an inspiration under which your own creativity will bloom. Art is a celebration of the life and world around us. Even in troubled times, and under less than ideal circumstances, art making can lift the spirit, communicate ideas and emotions, and offer new opportunities to grow and learn.

Explore your own creative self by delving more deeply into the interests you have, and the artwork and artists you enjoy. Release your fears and allow your ideas and skills to help others reach their potential.

Don't be afraid to embrace new technologies and to take the time to bring your clients into the new age with you. Generating beautiful artwork through many different media has never been easier, and even the least creative and most hesitant artist in each of us will find some means of self-expression. Providing the opportunity to express, explore, and extend one's self to others is a most valuable gift.

Most importantly, have fun and be fun. Seek out artistic opportunities in even the silliest or most unexpected places. Make the time you spend with your clients the highlight of their day, a place where they feel safe and cared for, and a refuge from troubles in their lives. Smile often and laugh frequently. Offer a welcoming, perhaps paint-stained, hand to the people around you and encourage them to join you in living a creative life.

Index

About the Author

Diane Fausek-Steinbach has been consulting or facilitating art therapy groups with long term care, rehabilitation, and general population clients for over 15 years and still reaches professionals through her quarterly “Brush Strokes” column in *Creative Forecasting Magazine.*

She has authored *The Practical Guide to Art Therapy Groups* (Fausek, Haworth Press, 1997), and *Art Activities for Groups: Providing Therapy, Fun, and Function* (Fausek-Steinbach, Idyll Arbor, 2002).

She continues to create meaningful art plans for a home schooling magazine and is currently a freelance writer in Iowa, where she lives with her husband and cat.